SUCCESS PRINCIPLES *of* Ratan Tata

VINOD SHARMA

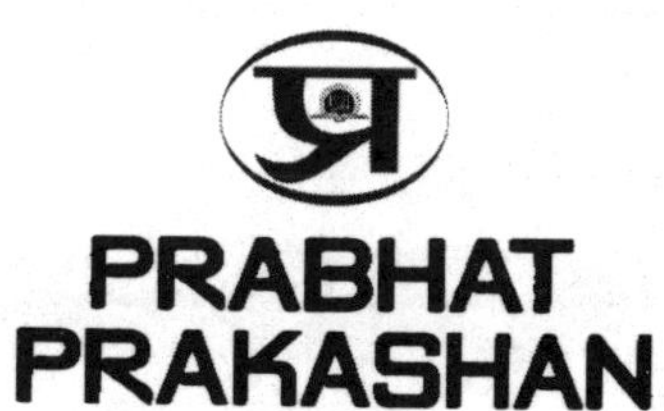

PRABHAT PRAKASHAN

Published by
PRABHAT PRAKASHAN PVT. LTD.
4/19 Asaf Ali Road,
New Delhi-110002 (INDIA)
e-mail: prabhatbooks@gmail.com

ISBN 978-93-5521-375-4
SUCCESS PRINCIPLES OF RATAN TATA
by Vinod Sharma

Edition
2026

Price
₹ 300 (Rupees Three Hundred Only)

Printed at
R-Tech Offset Printers, Delhi

Dedicated to the Vision & Wisdom of

Sir J.R.D. Tata

Author's Note

Sometimes the world is marked with the presence of certain personalities who remarkably contribute to society and the human race. Ratan Tata is one such individual whose success has not only inspired people throughout the Globe but has also given them an opportunity to make a better life for themselves. Success Principles of Ratan Tata tries to throw light on the life and achievements of Ratan Tata and how his life is a living example of diligence and modesty.

Ratan Tata's life inspires us in more than one way and the more we take a deeper look into his life, we are left amazed by his accomplishments. His innovative ideas and how he has shaped the legacy as per modern times is commendable and encouraging. Even though we can agree that he did inherit the Tata empire, his capabilities were never questionable. His strategies and ideas behind making the Tata company was unique. Unlike some businessmen he did not only want money, fame or success, he is also known for his philanthropy. The aim of Tata groups was not only their progress but also the progress of India. Ratan Tata did not always find a smooth road, he had his own hurdles and challenges but that did not stop him from achieving his goals.

The book caters to all groups and generations of people who are in need of some inspiration in their life. We can all look up to him for guidance and his life can be a lesson for us. We might not all want to be a businessman but his life is much more than that of a businessman. He brought glory and fame with hard work and has always remained true to his purpose. Ratan Tata is an extremely modest man holding good intentions for the society. We need more people like him for our country to grow and prosper in the right direction. He is also the role model for today's youth and he shall continue to be. Whatever was given to him was hereditary and he only added more to his family name and their purpose, keeping it uncorrupted and pure.

Anyone who wants to understand his life and workings can delve into this book and await their moment of amazement, epiphany and inspiration.

This can be life changing if one has the intention to do so. Ratan Tata's beliefs in humanity and benevolence shall always remain his root to the path of success.

❑

Contents

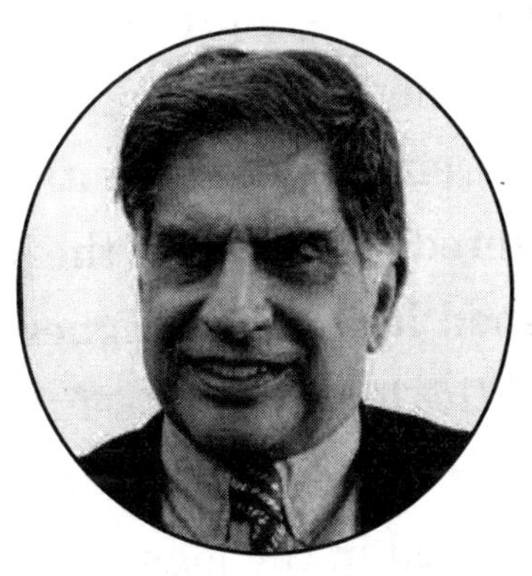

A Brief Note on Ratan Tata

The general notion of history teaches us that the success graph of a kingdom rises higher and after reaching a climax point, the glory tumbles down headlong. When an empire begins to be built, it becomes quite evident for the establisher to suggest innovative ideas and some ideologically superlative perspectives that can set a new throne up and strengthen it. But the continuation of the glory depends how the successors carry forward the legacy and maintain the balance right from the beginning. Though "Adversity always presents opportunities for introspection", some sort of dismissal happens from the hierarchical end, and the entire apartment is gradually shattered. If we look at the Mughal Empire, Babur established it with his highest power; Akbar carried forward the legacy successfully. But then the empire declined from several corners and points, and finally was destroyed in the long run.

But the exception of Tatas' managing business became quite a trademark in Indian history as it successfully carried forward the lineage without hampering the focused aim, though variably differed in different sectors. But from the days of Jamsetji Tata up to now, the Tatas consistently worked hard, thought and re-thought the process of making business superfluous with moderate improvisation and important modification. As history progresses, different 'leaders' appear and lead the monopoly with heavy responsibilities, thus strengthening the dynasty.

Ratan Tata is finally the one to be discussed and well-talked because of his amazing quality of understanding the public impulse, along with the contemporary societal study and political influence. He never failed to justify his forerunners perfectly, even when at the time of crisis, but dealt with every affair successfully, made their business to spread all over, and simultaneously opening some innovative corridors of ideas for the youth of India.

❑

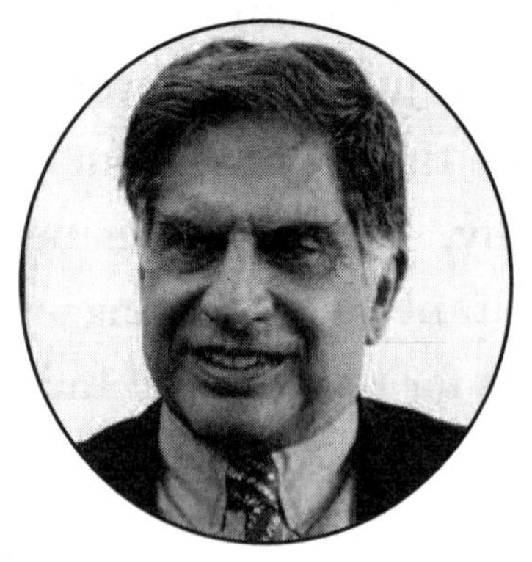

When the Baton Decides to Shift

It is back to one fine morning of 1991. The 87-year-old J.R.D. Tata had been the chairman of Tata for more than half a century. With the group's leading companies managed also by geriatric satraps, the last thing the Tata name stood for were flamboyance and energy; the more usual adjectives were staid and unenterprising. That was when a fairly young Ratan Tata (53) was selected as the group's new chairman, provoking questions about his performance (undistinguished) and so that of the capability, almost apart from the acceptability. Though the questions were answered long ago, but as usual, the acceptability was attained only by eliminating out some grey hairs. Two decades later, as a 75-year-old Ratan Tata planned to step down in 2012, the Tata group still stood for vibrancy, energy and enthusiasm to move forward, doing the business in typically the way Tata was known for. The monopoly never ended in Tata with just the absence of any household tycoon, as 44-year-old Cyrus Mistry took charge from then with a promising vibe. Tatas' working ethics and success principles were based on looking forward always with an innovative as well as daring (especially for the blue-prints overseas) ideas, along with tight shareholding and brand discipline. As Rahul Bajaj correctly remarked, Ratan Tata has changed the DNA – almost entirely for the better.

When India was opening up for globalization, liberalization and privatization in 1991, the iconic Tata group was pioneering a major organizational shake-up in terms of installing a non-committal Ratan Tata as successor of J.R.D. Tata. Indeed the top operation platoon working nearly with J.R.D. Tata had no indication about the transition. Also, Ratan Tata had no success stories that could inspire his elderly associates to accept him as the new chairman of the Tata Group. Still, no one had the guts to question the wisdom of J.R.D. Tata and therefore began the Ratan Tata period in the Tata Group.

The preliminary challenge for Ratan Tata was to establish his authority and increase effectiveness across the group companies which largely worked singly. For long, the Tata group companies had worked in a decentralized mode. But the decentralized arrangement deteriorated under the competitive forces that knocked at the doors of the country in the wake of opening up of the Indian economy at the decree of the International Monetary Fund and the World Bank. There could not have been a better and more intriguing time to take charge of the Tata Group for Ratan Tata "Who was at the right place at the right time and could see what was happening around him and respond accordingly". (Datta, 2012).

The group always finds options for amplifying its range, as it was 18 times bigger already than that of its width in 1991, if counted in US dollars; in rupees, it is 51 times bigger, and competed against successful tug-of-war with the rest of the corporate houses in India, dominating with highest appliance. The growth figures for gains are also fascinating. Both have been helped by the astral performance of Tata Consultancy Services (TCS), which remains the country's largest software services establishment. TCS also subsidized much of the increased intra-group shareholding and asset accession drives. But indeed without TCS, the group's performance under Ratan Tata has been phenomenal. Though growth in market capitalization (without TCS, which was listed only in 2004) has been below par at an annual rate of 10.8 per cent. The return on capital employed too has declined, from 15.2 per cent in 1992 to 14.4 per cent indeed with TCS — reflecting the below-rated performance of some of the overseas means, and the fact that an on-again-off-again Tata Motors has by far the smallest price-earnings multiple in the vehicle industry.

It is also important to note the particular quality with which Ratan Tata has conducted himself throughout these two dynamic and frequently tumultuous decades, and to admit that he long ago became the doyen of Indian industry. Sophisticatedly dressed, and moving calmly and quietly among the world's business tycoons, Mr. Tata has also acquired global standing for himself and his group — becoming, with ease, the largest private employer in the UK. Some would question his support of Narendra Modi when the Tata Nano project moved to Gujarat, others would point to the reproach at Tata Finance (led at the time by someone who had worked with Mr. Tata), and many will keep in mind Niira Radia and her formidable attempts to blow the choice of telecom minister in 2009. Mr. Tata has also had his run-sways with the media, repetitively denying words attributed to him, being most sensitive about criticism, and blacklisting one large media house after the other when it came to group advertising. But these are minor aspects of an impressive business career that in the end has more than justified J.R.D.'s choice of successor in 1991, and which leaves the Tata name shining brighter than the others.

❑

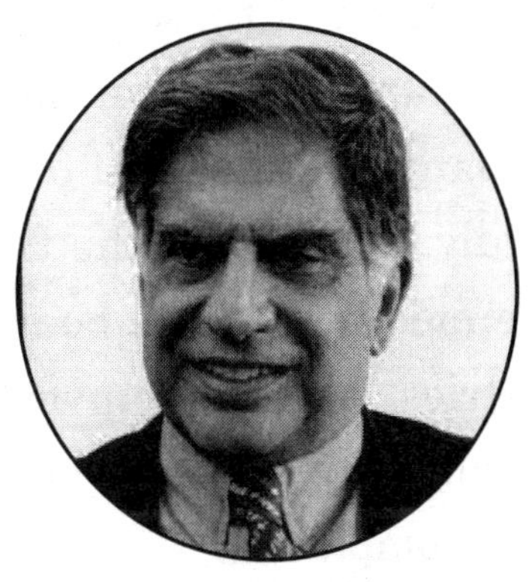

How the Legacy Continued to Rule

The Tata Group appeared in the scenario when Jamsetji Nusserwanji Tata started a trading establishment in 1868. The group set foot into manufacturing in 1874 (fabrics) and into services in 1904 (Hotels). Jamsetji's planning to advocate and set up new industries in the country was sustained by his son, Sir Dorabji Tata who succeeded him as the chairman of the group. He set up India's first steel factory in 1907, its first cement manufacturing unit in 1912 and the first indigenous insurance company in 1919. Each of these units was set up as an individual company. The Chairman of Tata Sons, the holding company and the chief protagonist of the group traditionally emerged as the Chairman of the Tata group. The members of the board of Tata Sons and Tata Industries, the other investment arms of the Group, are generally also members of the boards of different group companies.

Tata Group had always been avant-garde for the others of the contemporary time. And this pioneering spirit was not only limited to the world of business, but also propagated its zeitgeist to a broader extent. The group set up some of India's prestigious institutions – Indian Institute of Science, Tata Memorial Hospital, Tata Institute of Fundamental Research, Tata Institute of Social Sciences, Tata Energy Research Institute, and National Centre for Performing Arts. Jamsetji Tata said, "We do not claim to be more unselfish, more generous or more philanthropic than other people. But we think we started on sound principles, considering the interests of the shareholders our own, and the health and welfare of the employees, the sure foundation of our successive."

Lord Curzon, the then Viceroy of India, conceded the pioneering contribution of Jamsetji Tata. No other Indian, even today, has done better for the commercial trades and industry of India.

Jamsetji's sons, Sir Dorabji Tata, and Sir Ratanji Tata donated the utmost of their heritage and wealth for the welfare of the society when they established the Sir Dorabji Tata Trust and the Sir Ratan Tata Trust, independently. After Sir Dorabji's unfortunate death in 1932, Sir Nowroji Saklatwala, the third chairman of the group, continued the tradition of charity and donation for public welfare through several trusts. As a result, nearly two-thirds of the shares in Tata Sons are in custody of various charitable trusts. J.R.D. Tata (J.R.D.), who succeeded Saklatwala as the chairman of the group in 1938, explained, "The Tatas are in fact a trust and an institution more than just a business house. Right from the early days I knew Mahatma Gandhi and I was quite impressed and believed in the spirit of trusteeship ... I think that is the best way to apply the spirit of trusteeship – to act as trustees and to consider major problems of the country in connection with the firm as trustees and not as businessmen merely trying to make money for the firm. Incidentally, we want to make money because that is the only way to make funds available to charitable trusts".

JRD joined the Tata group in 1925 upon his father's urging, before he could complete his university education, prompting JRD to say, "Because of a lack of technical knowledge, my main contribution in management was to encourage others."

During the 52 times of JRD's leadership, the group entered varied businesses, growing from 14 companies in 1938 to a 95 company group in 1991, which included some of the flagship companies of the Group in 2016 – Tata Chemicals, Tata Motors, Tata Consultancy Services (TCS), Tata Tea and Titan Industries. While referring to the relationship between Tata Sons and its vividly associated companies, JRD had said, "I would call it a group of individually managed companies united by two factors ... that they are part of a larger group, the Tatas. Each company enjoys its share of privilege. Second, there is innate loyalty, a sharing of certain beliefs."

Over the times, to increase growth, JRD had allowed the dilution of Tata Sons' stake in the group companies performing in the group holding company having only a small, some would say emblematic, stake in the numerous group companies. In 1969, when the Government of India with a view to check the power of large business groups similar to the Tatas, introduced the Monopolies and Restrictive Trade Practices Act, the Tata group claimed that its cells were competently and resourcefully maintained by independent companies and J.R.D. was just a part-time chairman. J.R.D. said, "...Today, except in Tata Sons, I do not wield any kind of executive authority. But because I am senior in age, I operate more on the basis of influence and confidence."

Indeed when the non-supervisory restrictions were eased in the 1980s, J.R.D. Tata did not feel the need to institutionalize the group cooperation. Speaking to Tata group historian, R. M. Lala, J.R.D. elucidated his leadership style, "...with each man I have my own way. I am one who will make full allowance for a man's character and idiosyncrasies. You have to adapt yourself to their ways and deal accordingly and draw out the best in each man. One of the qualities of leadership is to assess what is needed to get the best results for an enterprise. If that demands being a very active executive chairman, as I was in Air India, I did that. On the other hand, in one of our other companies where I know that the managing director wishes to be alone and will get the results that way, it will be stupid for me to come in the way. At times, it involves suppressing yourself. It is painful but necessary ... To lead men; you have to lead them with affection."

Accordingly, CEOs of large Tata enterprises surfaced themselves as independent leaders in the Tata group. Tata experts—similar as—Darbari Seth, who played a crucial part in founding Tata Chemicals and Tata Tea, Ajit Kerkar who was necessary in promoting the Indian Hotels business, Tata Steel chairman Russi Mody, who successfully led the company through tough times, prestigious jurist Nani Palkhivala who was chairman of ACC Ltd. – emerged as important leaders in the Tata group. Kerkar observed, "He was the kind of chairman any professional manager should have. He laid down the policies but in no way interfered with the day-to-day working. ... He never imposed his own will on anything. That was his greatness".

During his term, JRD started group-wide enterprise similar to the Tata Administrative Services (TAS) to groom talented individuals for advanced operation careers in Tata companies, sustained Jamsetji's user-friendly ideologies by initiating various hand best-practices – an eight-hour working day, free medical aid, workers' provident scheme, and workmen's accident compensation schemes – that recently were made into law. For his social and entrepreneurial trials, J.R.D. Tata was awarded, India's loftiest mercenary honour, the Bharat Ratna, in 1992. He was the only businessman to have received the honour.

❑

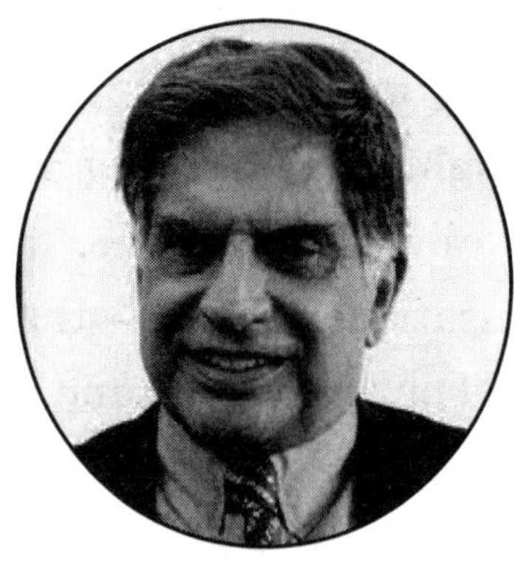

The New Captain: His Tournaments

Ratan Tata does not need any preface due to his fandom in trade-circles, for the group's achievements and being the most successful industrialist of India. He is popular in the launch-up circles for inspiring the youth through his life, ideology and especially the energy with which he capsized the failure of numerous companies to churn a profit, making the empire dazzlingly successful. The group has had great wealth which eventually has allowed it to grow by leaps and bounds in its continuance. He once commented that rise and fall is necessary in one's career as even the straight line in the ECG curve means lifelessness. He reminds the young generation that, to rise in the long run overcomes the short term failures.

He was born on December 28, 1937, in Surat, to Naval and Sonoo Tata. Naval Tata was the espoused son of Jamsetji Tata and Ratan Tata was raised by his paternal grandmother Lady Navajbai Tata after his parents' separation. Although they remained in contact, Ratan could not get the love, indulgence, support or the guidance from his own parents. He was close to his grandmother, who looked after him and raised him. She was a strict woman with a well-regulated approach to life and tasks.

Ratan Tata studied armature at Cornell University in the United States of America and had a job offer from IBM. Ratan Tata recollected, "I was quite happy with my work and, given a choice, I would have remained in the US". Still, he had to return to India in 1962, when Lady Navajbai's health deteriorated. Upon JRD's assignation, Ratan Tata joined the group and began his career 1962 as apprentice at the Jamshedpur factory of Tata Steel Ltd., also known as Tata Iron and Steel Company (TISCO). Over the coming 10 years, prior to being given the responsibility of turning around the ailing NELCO, Ratan Tata had stints in different group companies. Once, NELCO, one of the largest manufacturers of radios in the country, had lower than 3 per cent market shares and had significant accumulated losses when Ratan Tata took charge. Over the coming three years under his captainship, NELCO recovered achieving a market share of 20 per cent and taking back or retrieving its losses. Still in 1977, even though Ratan Tata believed in the abecedarian soundness of NELCO, the company was closed down owing to problems with the workers' union.

Soon after, Ratan Tata was given the responsibility to turn around Mumbai-grounded Empress Mills, yet another ailing company in the group. But his plans to contemporize the company did not receive the blessing of Tata Sons. He managed to energize the workers, but could not get acceptable backing support from the top management of Tata Group. Workers' strike worsened the script and eventually the Empress Mill was closed in 1986. Ratan Tata said, "At around this time, the whole Indian textile industry went through a bad patch. So, some Tata directors, chiefly Nani Palkhivala, took the line that we should liquidate the mill. I argued with them. We demanded just ₹50 lakhs (5 million) to turn it around. But Nani opposed giving us the money and we closed the mill down".

The experience with NELCO and Empress nudged Ratan Tata, a member of the panel of Tata Sons since 1974, to write to J.R.D. Tata about the need to have a strategic plan for the group, "I am strongly advocating the initiation of such a plan by the chairman as I personally see signs of our disintegration as a group. The first issue that needs to be addressed is whether we, as Tatas, see ourselves operating in the next 5 to 10 years as a single unified group, or a loosely connected agglomeration of independent companies ... If at all it is decided that the Tatas should operate as a group, then several strategic decisions need to be taken relating to the projected organizational and operational structure of the Tatas." Ratan Tata recalled, "I used to discuss the matter with JRD, why don't we find a mechanism to pull ourselves together? At that time, I was looking at a logo – not the new one – and was asking why don't we use that as glue and demand things from companies and give things to companies. But he never really supported that because he felt that it was not necessary. And from his standpoint, he was the patriarch, they were his team and there was no need to do all this."

In 1983, soon after he was appointed the chairman of Tata Industries, Ratan Tata progressed with a group-wide strategic plan, which proposed the invention of the newest technology supports, adding the group's transnational business and moving out of underperforming businesses. The plan also suggested that the group companies cash in on the group's size and variety and stressed making Tata a more unified structure through increased power. Tata Industries, which after the rescinding of the managing agency system had been without a clear accreditation, came as the group's vehicle for entry into the proposed new businesses. Fresh equity infusion from group companies – Tata Steel, Tata Motors, Indian Hotels Co., Tata Oil Mills Co., Tata Chemicals, and Voltas – evolved in Tata Industries pursuing several of the recently linked openings.

More recently, following his appointment as Chairman of Tata Motors, Ratan Tata encouraged the company to expand its portfolio. Tata Motors first entered the mileage vehicles segment with the launch of Tata Sumo and followed it up by entering into a common adventure with Mercedes Benz to assemble cars for trade in India and explore the capability for exports.

Ratan Tata's engagement as chairman of the group coincided with the liberalization of the Indian economy, which radically changed India's commercial topography. The steering in of global competition urged several people to prognosticate that Indian companies after having operated in a secured economy for decades would lose out to new and nimble competition. The Tata group was considered particularly vulnerable due to its size, diversity, decentralized structure, and therefore the recent retirement of its long serving chairman, J.R.D. Tata. Ratan Tata agreed saying, "I think the group needed cohesion, or let me put that another way, the cohesion the group had was through the persona of J.R.D. Tata, the patriarch. My concern was that after him, it would be difficult to hold it together."

❑

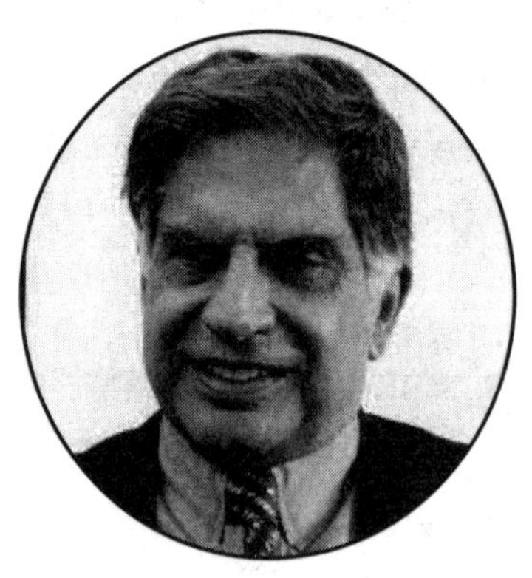

The Tycoon Typhoon

In the 1980s when JRD started considering his choice of the next heir, interposers at the Tata group thought that Russi Mody would succeed him. Ratan Tata said, "For most of the 1980s, I personally thought that Russi was certain to be the next head of Tatas. He ran Tata Steel very successfully, had a larger-than-life personality and Jeh (JRD) was very fond of him. Russi was gregarious. He was outgoing. He could go into a crowd of workers and charm them."

In 1988, JRD asked Russi Mody to also head Tata Motors. Still, when Russi Mody spoke disparagingly about Tata Motors to the press, the also Tata Motors' chairman, Sumant Moolgaonkar refused to hand over charge to Mody and sought the appointment of Ratan Tata as the company's chairman. Later, in March 1991, when JRD declared the comparatively less known and reticent Ratan Tata as his successor, it caused unusual drama and displeasure within the group. Unlike the opposite contenders for the position, Ratan Tata had no displayable success till even the two Tata companies that he headed ahead, NELCO and Empress Mills had folded up. Remembering his initial days, Ratan Tata stated, "J.R.D. Tata had around him a team of senior managers, all of them people of substantial understanding in their respective spheres. While they may have acceded to his wish that I take over the chairmanship – and this happened suddenly – I must confess that I did not feel any sense of joyousness on their part, because some of them had aspirations to have the job themselves."

Ratan Tata's concerns about the group's outlook stemmed to some extent from the structural tribulations that he encountered as a chairman. He had little control over the companies because of the low ownership stakes that Tata Sons held in them. Also, during the 53 years of JRD's tenure of chairmanship, the chieftains of group companies had total freedom with little authorial countersign and that they made it clear that they wished to protect their respective fields. Darbari Seth, Chairman of Tata Chemicals and Tata Tea, put it bluntly, "The Tata group is a commonwealth of enterprises, not an empire".

Ratan Tata had his first battle with Russi Mody when the second appointed Aditya Kashyap, his protégé, as joint managing director, without the permission of the company's board. Only after JRD's intervention and multiple conversations with the board did Mody withdraw his decision.

The two got further in moral combat when in early 1992 Ratan Tata revived an old policy that set the retirement age for administrative directors (including managing directors and executive chairmen) at 65 years and for non-executive directors at 75 years. Mody, 74 years at that time, complied by giving up his administrative position and continued as the non-executive chairman of Tata Steel. Still, before he was to retire fully from Tata Steel, his conflict with the Tata Steel board and Ratan Tata boosted, frequently in the public sphere. An agonized Ratan Tata said, "I don't understand why Russi behaved the way he did. He was my friend. He was Jeh's favourite. But he just became totally unreasonable. I remember one board meeting where we asked him why he kept giving interviews running down Tata Steel, of which he was the chairman. (J.J. Irani was MD.) He just got up and said, 'I will leave the room because this subject has been raised.' And then, to our astonishment, the chairman of Tata Steel got up and walked out of his own board meeting. After that he didn't turn up for board meetings and kept maligning the company. Finally, the board had to remove him."

The unfortunate competitiveness of the two flagship companies of the group Tata Steel and Tata Motors, of which he was now the chairman, was the second most important challenge for Ratan Tata. Years of leadership, achieved in an unrestricted frugality isolated from serious competition, had rendered these companies with an organizational culture that had scant regard for cost, quality, or client satisfaction. Presumably in the changed environment, both the companies, which constituted 50 per cent of the group's development, faced a severe decline in their earnings and profits in 1992. Ratan Tata set about transubstantiating them. He said, "I made no effort to play a group part until TISCO and TELCO were doing extremely well."

Apart from concentrating on the three crucial motorists of competitiveness, he made significant investments in upgrading their technology and revamping their product portfolio. While Tata Steel increased the share of value-added products in its client immolations, Tata Motors blazoned its plans to produce an indigenously developed passenger car, Indica. Still, the company's plans to incursion into passenger cars met with dubitation. Judges considered the move veritably parlous as the company, basically a manufacturer of marketable vehicles, had no experience in designing cars. The venture if it failed could ruin the company. Ratan Tata did not agree, "I think risk is a necessary part of business philosophy. You can be risk-averse and take no risks, in which case you will have a certain trajectory in terms of your growth. Or you can, while being prudent, take a greater risk in order to grow faster. I think, as a group, we were risk-averse and we hardly grew because either it was not safe or no one else had done it ahead. I view risk as an ability to be where no one has been before. I view risk to be an issue of thinking big, something we did not do previously. We did everything in small increments so we always lagged behind."

Over the next two years, the advancements in quality and productivity resulted in both companies' recording significant advancements in their performance. Indeed, while helping the flagship companies ameliorate performance, in order to grab the new openings made available by profitable reforms, Ratan Tata entered into collaborations with multinationals and set up several high technology foundations such as Tata Teleservices (Bell Canada) and Tata Communications in the telecom sector, Tata Petrodyne in upstream oil and gas (with BP), Tata Information Systems in information technology (with IBM) and initiated conversations with Singapore Airlines to launch airline services in India. To fund the new initiatives, Ratan Tata vended 20 per cent stakes in Tata Industries Ltd. to the Hong Kong grounded Jardine Matheson group for $35 million (Rs. 1.26 billion).

As a primary step towards integrating and getting the different cells to favour support a group, Ratan Tata sought to extend Tata Sons' stake within the group companies. Tata Sons made a rights issue of equity shares for ₹3 billion and the different trusts renounced their rights in favour of the group companies who subscribed to the equity. The fund therefore raised was used to increase the stake in group companies. Ratan Tata explained, "There was a question whether we had the right to claim to manage these companies. In fact we didn't have the legal right, or even the moral right, to manage them. Then we set ourselves the task of seeing how we could put ourselves together as a more meaningful and recognizable group of companies with more central control."

Organizing the different businesses into a coherent structure came next. With the help of the consulting establishment, McKinsey & Company, Ratan Tata organized the various businesses into seven sectors — information technology and communications, engineering products and services, accoutrements, services, energy, consumer products, and chemicals.

Many of the cells had overlapping businesses—ACC, Tata Chemicals, and TISCO made cement; Merind and Tata Pharma had presence in the medicinal field. These businesses were moreover consolidated into one of the cells or vended. Ratan Tata elaborated, "The kind of structural change that we are seeking is giving more attention to performance and measurement of performance, greater mobility between companies in terms of manpower and a greater focus in companies on strategic issues rather than on tactical operations."

Along with the reformation, Ratan Tata started enterprises to strengthen the group's cohesion. In 1998, he introduced the Tata Brand Equity and Business Promotion Agreement between Tata Sons and the group companies. The agreement quested that Tata Sons, the proprietor of the Tata name and brand totem, would promote the group brand and cover the interests of the group companies, both in India and worldwide. The Tata brand name itself was to be worn with significant concern. If an undertaking company fell outside the core businesses of the group or was perceived as a parlous new adventure where the group had limited experience, the Tata name was not used. One such company was Trent, the retail venture, started by Simone Tata, following the trade of Lakme to the Unilever subsidiary in India, Hindustan Unilever.

Though the agreement was not obligatory, companies that wanted to use the Tata name were needed to take part in the programme by paying an annual figure to Tata Sons. The Tata Brand Equity agreement divided the companies into two categories – companies that used the Tata name directly, and had a strong association with the Tata name; and companies that did not use the Tata name directly. With an intention to produce single strong equity that would profit all the companies, it was proposed that the first tier companies would contribute 0.25 per cent of development, or 5 per cent of profit before duty, whichever was less. Further, the other pealed companies would contribute 0.15 per cent of the development. Ratan Tata said, "If you are to fight a Mitsubishi or an X or Y in the free India of tomorrow, you better have one rather than 40 brands. You better have the ability to promote that brand in a meaningful manner."

The tax of brand figure was explosively blamed by the old bureaucrats and critics. Nani Palkhivala, the then chairman of ACC, affirmed that while ACC was an associate of the group, it was not a Tata Group company. Ajit Kerkar, chairman and managing director of Indian Hotels argued the company had no way used the Tata name and hence did not owe a figure to Tata Sons. Echoing these sentiments, the well-known columnist Swaminathan Aiyar wrote, “So many Tata branded products have flopped that the Tata brand is by no means a winner. The group’s textile mills and Tata Oil fell sick; Lakme was sold before it suffered a similar fate. Titan Watches and Indian Hotels have prospered but neither carries the Tata name ... TISCO and TELCO have created the Tata reputation and cynics will say they should demand money from Ratan Tata for giving his name similar prestige and not the other way around.”

Ratan Tata in defence observed “When a company would go to its bankers, it was part of the Tata group; when it went to seek a new collaboration, the literature spent a long time talking about the Tata group of which it was a part. But, after those situations that had been achieved the issue of being a member of the Tata group sort of slipped into a lower grade."

Signatories to the brand contract were needed to pledge the Tata Code of Conduct that codified the group's translucent and moral business practices. They also demanded to meet with certain performance conditions, which included being among the top three in their separate industries, double their turnover every four years and, profit after tax every three years. Ratan Tata said, "Over the years we didn't standard ourselves against the best of the breed, either in India or globally. Some companies never looked at market share, and we always compared ourselves traditionally to our past ... many of them got into the phase of reacting to the market rather than being proactive."

In December 1998, seven of the Tata companies—TISCO, TELCO, Tata Tea, Tata Chemicals, the Tata Electric Companies, Tata International, and Tata Industries—signed the agreement. To make the Tata name more prominent and suggestive of the Tata connection to its companies in the minds of the stakeholders, TISCO was renamed as Tata Steel and TELCO appeared as Tata Motors. The different ensigns used by group companies were also replaced with a common group totem.

To help him oversee the restructuring sweats, Ratan Tata found a five-member group administrative office (GEO). The members were N.A. Soonawala, Director of Tata Sons, R. Gopalakrishnan (Executive Director, Tata Sons), Ishaat Hussain (Executive Director, Finance, TISCO and later, Director, Finance, Tata Sons), Kishore Chaukar (Managing Director, Tata Industries Limited) and Manab Bose (Director, Human Resources, Tata Group). The GEO was a companion to group companies in strategic planning, benchmarking performance, and in allocating assets. To oversee performance and to enhance the commerce between the superintendents of the affiliated companies and Tata Sons, the GEO set up Business Review Panels (BRC) for each of the cells. The panels comported of representatives from Tata Sons and external agencies such as financial institutions. Ratan Tata noted "The BRC is not focusing on what is necessary for the Tata group ... It is not an internal Tata board, it is a committee of the company's board ... The BRC focuses on trying to make a company more profitable, more productive ... In fact, the directors of the companies were concerned that this would take away the autonomy of the board. It is not so. The BRC will, in fact, eventually make its recommendation to the board through this board committee and the board will finally take its decision."

To help companies identify areas of betterment, the Tata Business Excellence Model (TBEM) was introduced. The TBEM, which was modeled along the lines of the Malcolm Balridge National Quality Award, set a brand for all Tata companies all through seven core aspects of business operations: leadership, strategic planning, client focus, dimension, analysis and knowledge operation, workforce focus, process operation and issues of fiscal and non-financial parameters, and business results. The JRD Quality Value award was to be given to the company that scored the highest on the benchmarking.

Tata Motors launched Indica which got rave reviews for its design and comfort. Still soon, client complaints about the product quality and machine performance started coming in. Deals did not go as anticipated. Tata Motors reported a net loss of ₹5 billion because of the commuter auto blueprint, the biggest loss posted by any private sector company in India and the highest loss in the history of the Tata group. The company improved its gains by following the TBEM recommendations of quality enhancement, cost reduction, re-engineering of processes, and new product development. Also, Tata Steel embraced TBEM recommendations to come out as one of the smallest cost manufacturers of steel in the world and aligned its product processes to market dynamics. The company brought down its per-ton cost of product from $225 to $150, the second lowest worldwide. B Muthuraman, Managing Director, Tata Steel, asserted, "With all these sweats, Tata Steel, by the year 2001, had become one of the lowest cost producers of steel in the world and began to be recognized in the global steel industry. We had earned the right to grow."

In 2002, Ratan Tata founded the Group Corporate Centre (GCC), initially consisted of himself and other senior group executives – N.A. Soonawala, R.K. Krishna Kumar and J.J. Irani - to give premeditated track and escalation openings to the group companies and made the GEO its managerial arm. To patron the expansion of the group, Tata Sons made TCS public. The group vended 13 stakes in the company for $1.2 billion (Rs. 54.2 billion). Ratan Tata said, "The proceeds from the IPO will be used to help the Tata group continue restructuring its balance sheet, promoting new ventures, and deepening its involvement in existing group companies."

Companies responded to Ratan Tata's call for promoting new initiatives by bearing several new systems. In the marketable vehicle section, Tata Motors could relate the need for a four-wheeled vehicle that could serve as a last-afar distribution transport. For ferrying goods over small distances there were either exchanges, which were expensive or there were three-wheeled auto cabs that were unsafe and energy hamstrung. The company launched Tata Ace in 2005 that was priced on par with three-wheeler auto-rickshaws but had the cargo capacities of a four-wheeler truck and importantly, handled safety and maneuverability suitable to Indian roads. The product was a moment megahit.

In the new technology areas, the group established presence altogether aspects of telecom services – land-line and wireless services employing CDMA technology through Tata Telecom, GSM cellular services through collaboration with AT&T and Birlas, long distance calling, internet and value-added services through Tata Communications, following the accession of state-possessed company Videsh Sanchar Nigam Limited.

In the technology business, with a view to globalize its footmark, Tata Tea sought to acquire Tetley, the UK-grounded global tea major. The company's $318 million shot failed as it could not put together its backing arrangements well in time. R.K. Krishna Kumar, Managing Director of Tata Tea at that time recalled, "We realized that we had to get our act together on our funding arrangements well in advance, if we ever desired to make such a large global acquisition. It was a lesson well learnt."

In 2000, when Tetley came up for trade again, Tata Tea bid $435 million and won. The preemption was the group's first transnational accession and the largest cross-border preemption by an Indian company at that time. Tata Tea, which was a third of the size of Tetley beat competition from US consumer products major Sara Lee and Nestle, the Swiss foods major and surfaced as the world's second largest tea company with deals in 44 countries. Ratan Tata affirmed, "In a world where brand strength is crucial, the acquisition of Tetley will give Tata Tea a global opportunity."

The deal was substantially financed through a debt of $320 million, and as a consequence, Tetley continued to function as an "independent" company with Tata Tea playing largely a monitoring part. Homi Khusrokhan, the then managing director of Tata Tea, said, "A leveraged buy-out has perforce certain limitations attached to it, in terms of what you can and can't do as long as the high leverage continues. Therefore, in the early days following the acquisition, Tata Tea restricted its role to an advisory one: monitoring, guiding and watching over Tetley's operations."

After two years, Tata Tea and Tata Sons raised their stake in the company, released high cost debt, and integrated Tetley's operations to capture solidarity in areas of tea buying and blending.

The Tetley accession was the launch of the globalization drive at the Tata Group. The Group

Centre signed Alan Rosling from Jardine Matheson to forefront the operation and Arun Gandhi, a leading chartered accountant, who had advised Tata Tea in the Tetley accession to give the necessary valuation and taxation moxie. Ratan Tata said, "I have felt for some time that we have been an inward looking group. We could have gone overseas much earlier; the Aditya Birla Group did that many years ago. But we were obsessed with ourselves in India. And I suddenly felt – certainly when I started to sit on boards overseas — very conspicuous by the fact that we were only in India".

Over the coming decade, the Tata Group companies made a string of accessions. Affiliated companies linked targets that either filled gaps in their product portfolios or handed sourcing advantages or gave access to new geographical markets. The GCC handed M&A premonitory support, helped the group companies to unite capital, assessed whether the target company would fit into the Tata's values and handed post-acquisition integration support. Importantly, it acted as a repository of knowledge and moxie transferring literacy from former accessions to the affiliated cells.

Speaking of its accession of Daewoo Commercial Vehicle Company in Korea, Ravi Kant, and Vice Chairman of Tata Motors said, "Tata Motors was one of ten bidders, including Chinese and European companies. Initially, we faced some difficulty in being accepted as a serious bidder. I think the one thing that helped us win the deal was our philosophy. Mr. Ratan Tata suggested that we should see ourselves as a Korean company, not as an Indian company in Korea. That made all the difference."

In the starting quarter of 2007, Tata Motors acquired the ailing decoration luxury car brand Jaguar and top of the line mileage vehicle brand Land Rover from Ford Motor Company for roughly $2.3 billion. Though Tata Motors intended to buy only the Land Rover, Ford was selling both the brands (JLR) as a combo. The GCC helped Tata Motors raise the $3 billion (about ₹120 billion) from multiple banks. Critics and investors said Tata Motors was making a huge mistake, especially since experienced car makers similar to BMW and Ford could not turn around JLR. Still, Ratan Tata saw it as a unique occasion to move into prime section with access to world class iconic brands. Ravi Kant said, "The deal has dramatically changed the perception of Tata Motors worldwide. People see us differently now, with greater respect. Doors that were closed earlier are now opening. People are coming on their own from all corners of the world and making so many offers. It created a great impact."

The economic crisis occurred soon after the deal closed, and demand for luxury cars tumbled in Europe and North America — its two biggest markets. Tata Motors posted a loss of $520 million in financial year 2009. Analysts were not so astonished; they were rather out in droves with their "we told you so" reports. Undeterred, the company indeed as it embarked on a serious cost reduction action, explored new market deals in other countries, like China, Saudi Arabia, Russia, etc. By 2010, JLR turned profitable and soon came the dependence of Tata Motors in terms of both earnings and gains.

Still, JLR was not Tata group's biggest accession to date. Towards the end of 2006, Tata Steel acquired British Steel maker, Corus for $12.1 billion, following a competitive bidding process. Tata Steel had gained experience in acquiring Natsteel in Singapore and

Millennium Steel in Thailand that strengthened its resource chain and handed access to East Asian markets. The company had originally bid $7.6 billion for Corus, which was challenged by CSN, a Brazilian steel company. The ensuing months observe extreme negotiations from both sides of the deal. Eventually, in January 2007, Tata Steel bought a 100 per cent stake in the Corus. The deal, by far the largest overseas attainment any Indian company made Tata Steel the world's fifth-largest steel patron, with an annual aptitude of 25 million tons.

As in the case of JLR, the 2008 recession deeply impacted Corus. Several changes in the top operation circuit, slow amalgamation of the company by Tata Steel compounded the challenges and as a result, Corus, a profit-making company at the time of its succession, went astray by $303 million in 2010. While the company managed to turn around the very coming year, following job cuts and asset trade, the debt-laden company was still floundering to ameliorate the performance of its European operations.

While the Tata companies were making rapid strides in international markets with accessions, near home they were developing affordable products that served the lower income zones. Ratan Tata said, "All along, the focus of entrepreneurs and corporations has been to develop products for the top of the pyramid that has about 250-300 million people. Though these people constitute about 25-30 per cent of the population, the need of the hour is to create products and services for the remaining 1.2 billion Indians."

One of the successful inventions from the Tata group was Tata Swach, the world's cheapest water cleaner. Access to clean drinking water has been hectic in most Indian villages, small towns, and semi-urban locales and in matrices of civic areas. Tata group set out to find a market-based result to give clean drinking water and reduce health problems arising from drinking polluted water. As a result of collaboration among TCS, Tata Chemicals and Titan Industries, the Swach technology combined low-cost constituents such as rice cocoon ash with superior nanotechnology. It does not need electricity or running water to operate and meets international water sanctification norms. Its affordable price – ₹500, ₹750 and ₹1000 for three variants – put the product within the reach of consumers at the bottom of the social class.

As chairman of the Tata Group, Ratan Tata concentrated on accelerating functional effectiveness and culture of invention which was all the more important in the wake of increased competitiveness in the country, rising foreign direct investments in nearly all the sectors and changing prospects of the stakeholders. Interventions at the decree of Ratan Tata enabled Tata Steel Ltd. to become the smallest cost steel makers of the world (Datta, 2012). Likewise, significant advancements were witnessed in Tata Motors Ltd. as well.

Ratan Tata strictly strengthened the authority of Tata Sons Ltd. – The holding company of all the Tata Group companies by adding the stakes. Before, Tata Sons Ltd. had non-age stakes in most of the Group companies which made them vulnerable to hostile appropriations. Also, he introduced the system of gross payment by the Group companies for using the Tata brand name. This enhanced the brand equity of Tata Group presently.

Some of the less profitable businesses such as cement, fabrics and cosmetics under the marquee of Tata Group were dropped under the leadership of Ratan Tata. On the other hand, he entered the rising areas such as software, telecommunication, finance and retail. Either, Ratan Tata's major benefactions would include global accessions similar to Tetley Tea, Corus Group, and Jaguar Land Rover.

Ratan Tata is credited with massive financial success during his term as Chairman of the Group. The Group's total deals at the end of 2011-12, at ₹4.51 trillion, was 43 times the development in 1992-93, the first full financial achievement after Tata took over as chairman; while net profit growth in the same period was indeed more spectacular, rising 51 times (Datta, 2012). Also, the entire market capitalization of the group at ₹4.54 trillion in financial years of 2012-13 is 33 times superior than it had been in 1992-93. In the same period, the Sensex, the standard equity indicator of BSE, grew nearly eight times' (Datta, 2012). Still, one of the most precious failures of the Tata Group was Tata Nano – a public car that Ratan Tata promoted despite resistance from within the group.

The Tata Nano was the extreme major action accepted by the group following the observation of Ratan Tata that Indian families that could not enjoy a car demanded a safe and affordable four-wheeler transport. In 2003 at the Geneva Auto Show, Ratan Tata blazoned that the company would develop a people's car that would be priced at $2500. The advertisement attracted transnational attention and the ultra-low-cost car ingrained Nano appeared as the most talked-about car, as world over, people waited for its release. The excitement still did not result in deals when the car was launched in 2009. Ratan Tata said, "The Nano is something I would love to make successful because I don't suppose it has exploited its full potential right now. There has to be another push to make Nano what it can be."

Tata Group Innovation Forum (TGIF) was set up to promote invention. To increase exchange of ideas and learning, TGIF operated a platform, Innoverse, which enabled members to seek results to new problems. Further, to fete the invention efforts of the different group companies, TGIF organized a yearly invention competition entitled - Innovista.

❑

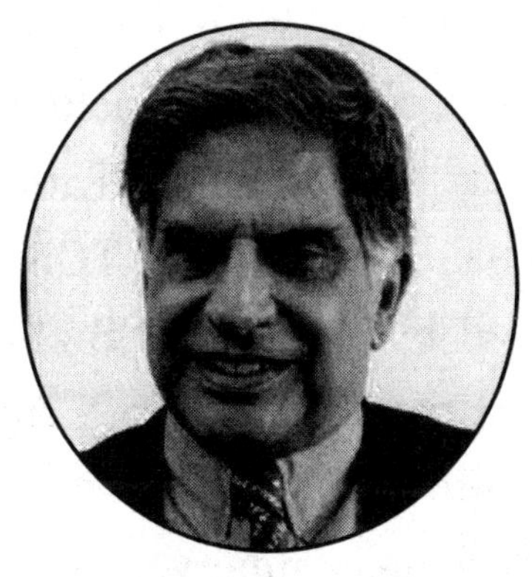

TCS and Tata: The Bosom Friendship

Apart from his vision, what helped Ratan Tata pursue his global dreams was the extraordinary success of Tata Consultancy Services, which are 74 per cent possessed by Tata Sons. Beginning with its preliminary public immolation in August 2004, which helped Tata Sons rise to around 2,800 crores; TCS laterally funded the bulk of investments by Tata Sons in major group companies as they sought to conquer the worldwide business of technological matrix. The figures speak for themselves. Since 2004, Tata Sons has invested a bulk amount of ₹34,000 crores in different group companies, including unrecorded gambles. During the period, Tata Sons earned nearly ₹10,000 as dividend from TCS; another ₹9100 crores was raised by dealing TCS shares (including IPO). Again, ₹11,500 crores came from borrowings essentially secured by pledging shares of TCS, the group's most precious company.

So, if not for TCS, Tata might have had to either gauge down his global intentions or the backing cost of big-ticket global accessions would have stretched the group's balance sheet to an unsustainable situations. Investment bankers agree. "The majority control of TCS gives great financial firepower to Tata Sons. The recurring cash from TCS and the market value of TCS provided Tata Sons the cushion to absorb minor losses if the bet didn't work out in the short term," said, Dara Kalyaniwal, vice-president, investment banking, at Prabhudas Lilladher. He is not exaggerating. Tata Sons' wager in TCS is currently valued at around ₹1.8

lakh crores, almost six per cent of which was pledged at the end of September. In comparison, Tata Sons' holding in all listed group companies is presently valued at around Rs 2.4 lakh crores.

TCS has a policy to distribute 30-50 per cent of net profit as dividends, in four quarterly transactions. In FY 2010, still, it distributed 55 per cent of consolidated net profit and 70 per cent of its standalone net profit as equity dividend, by way of a special dividend. Ratings agencies honour the power of TCS, which, they say, plays a significant part in Tata Sons getting overwhelming AAA ratings, helping it to adopt at the smallest possible rate of interest. "The ratings reflect Tata Sons' exceptional financial flexibility which arises from its ability to raise additional funds by sell or pledge of TCS shares," said CRISIL, while assigning top standing to Tata Sons' non-convertible debenture programme in November.

Icra holds an analogous view. "AAA ratings incorporate Tata Sons' strong financial flexibility despite increase in the debt levels to support the funding requirement of its investee companies," said the agency.

The group's globalization drive and its craving for inorganic growth have nearly followed the augmentation of TCS within the last ten years. And, as TCS got larger, so did the aspiration of its chairman. The holding company has dashingly leveraged the newer cash overflows from TCS (as dividends) to adopt and support different group growth plans.

A harmonious fiscal performance by TCS and its high market valuation enabled Tata Sons to act as the investor and lender of last resort to group companies. For instance, when Tata Motors' business rights issue in October 2008 regressed on promoters and Indian Hotels Company's rights issue in 2008 entered muted response from retail and institutional investors. TCS also enabled Tata to see new businesses and nearly half the Tata Sons portfolio is reckoned for by its investment in unrecorded accessories.

As of now, there is no sign of any retardation in the TCS cash machine. In the first half of the FY 2012, net profit rose to 43 per cent, while earnings were over by 36 per cent on a consolidated base. This has restated into handsome earnings for shareholders, including Tata Sons, which has formerly received ₹3,175 crores in the first six months, 30 per cent more than what it earned during the whole of FY 2012. More is waiting to come in the last quarter.

❑

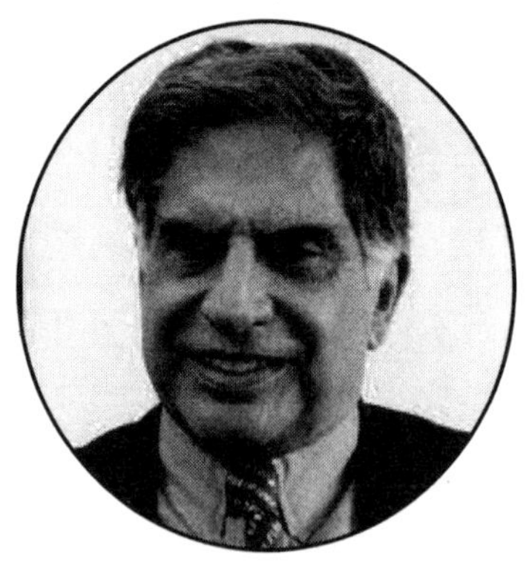

When the Cacophony Sounds Melodious

At a dinner party in Taj Chambers on July 22, 1993, after a lengthy annual general meeting of Tata Steel, Ratan Tata asked B. Muthuraman and T. Mukherjee (elderly general managers then), "Would you let the bluest of blue chip companies have a red bottom line?" The reference of that question was a miserable first quarter result within the background of competition from imports, indicating a transition to a buyer's market. The question helped Tata, who was then new to his post of Tata Steel chairman, prize a pledge from the two gentlemen. Before the end of the financial year, the company would reduce cost by Rs 500 a ton, which restated to 7.5 per cent of the cost at that point in time. Till that time, every year cost had gradually risen.

By December, at a meeting that lasted till two in the morning, Tata was told by a group of veritably satisfied executives that they had managed a cost reduction of ₹350 a ton.

But Tata's reply was a clear sign of dissatisfaction, "Your promise is with me, you don't have to make another promise. What's at stake is your prestige and reputation."

The comment was, thus, loud and clear. By March, costs were reduced by ₹500 a ton indeed, though there was an increase on nearly every other count, including railway freight. Target-led invention had made it possible.

It was an achievement indeed, but towards the late 1990s, profitability started suffering again, urging Tata Steel to appoint three advisers — Booze Allen

Hamilton, McKinsey and Arthur D' Little. The report sheet: a grade 'C'.

Tata Steel was told in clear terms that it was inadequate and no good compared to global peers. McKinsey had indeed advised that the steel business was subject to commodity cycles and Tata Steel should diversify.

It came as a rude jolt, but the operation took the cue. From 1995 to 2001, Tata Steel reduced work-power from 78,300 to 47,300 by enforcing a voluntary withdrawal scheme (VRS), and an early separation scheme (ESS). At the administrative position, Tata Steel introduced the performance ethic programme. Had the VRS not been introduced in 1995, all its gains, especially in 2001-02, would have gone towards payment of hires. In a nutshell, Tata Steel would have been in the red.

But the company bounced back. In 2001, it stood first in the World Steel Dynamics (WSD) list of world class steel makers against several parameters that included operating cost, technology, product quality, position in the domestic market.

Small accessions — NatSteel and Millennium Steel — followed and till 2006, that is before Tata

Steel acquired Corus, the company featured among the top four steel makers in the world. But following two financial turmoil states that resounded through the world, Tata Steel has slid down the list. A lot of it is connected to its European operations.

Five years after the high profile buyout of Corus — the biggest foreign accession made by an Indian company at $12 billion in those times — Tata Steel is at a crossroads. At 608 pence a share, the price was a 34 per cent premium to Tata Steel's actual offer. Though the deal pelted Tata Steel to the fifth largest steel maker, in hindsight, it looks like an expensive deal.

The Tata Steel group's fortunes have seesawed with steel prices, primarily because the European operations that regard for 60 per cent of earnings do not have locked up raw material coffers, unlike its Indian operations. Jointly, coking coal and iron ore, account for about 65 per cent of the total cost of steel production. Naturally, profitability has slipped over the years. From an enormous amount of ₹12,322 crores at the end of March 2008, Tata Steel's net profit after tax reduction stood at ₹449 crores in 2009 and in 2010 it suffered a loss of ₹2,121 crores. The year 2011 was finally better, worth ₹8,856 crores; but again it declined in 2012, and the price was almost halved to ₹4,949 crores.

Raw ingredients, however, are still a part of the bigger problem. According to some, Corus buys the Rolls-Royce of raw accessories, but with that it is possible to attain records in specific parameters, not gains. It is a combination of factors that affects Tata Steel Europe, raw material apart, similar as under-investment implantations by quondam promoters, and high hand cost, though Tata Steel has lowered significantly, and retardation in Europe.

There are issues with the integration process as well. Ratan Tata had lately said the former British managers of Corus were not prepared to go the extra mile. Whether that has affected the $450 million savings from unification anticipated to be achieved over three years is not known.

Of course, some interned raw material will flow in from Riversdale. Tata Steel is anticipated to receive its first payload of 850,000 tons of coking coal and 200,000 tons of thermal coal from these mines in Mozambique shortly. But for its European operations that have a capacity of about 18 million tons yearly, it could just be a drop in the ocean.

The demand script for Corus does not seen relatively bright either, at least in the near future. According to Tata Steel's assumption, the European economy was believed to contract in 2012, with only borderline growth predicted in 2013. That is not encouraging news for a company which now depends on Europe for 66 per cent of its total product capacity.

So, the focus obviously would be to correct the imbalance and concentrate on India to achieve business growth. The Indian operations are on a steady course, which is poised to grow more once the steel factory at Kaliganagar is commissioned in 2014, though the curriculum is delayed by about five years and Tata Steel is almost sure to miss its target of achieving a capacity of 50 million tons by 2015.

Recently, Ratan Tata observed in his interview to the groups' in-house journal that his involvement in Tata Steel's growth and elaboration has been significant. It appears that his successor will have a lot to unbend in the group flagship.

❑

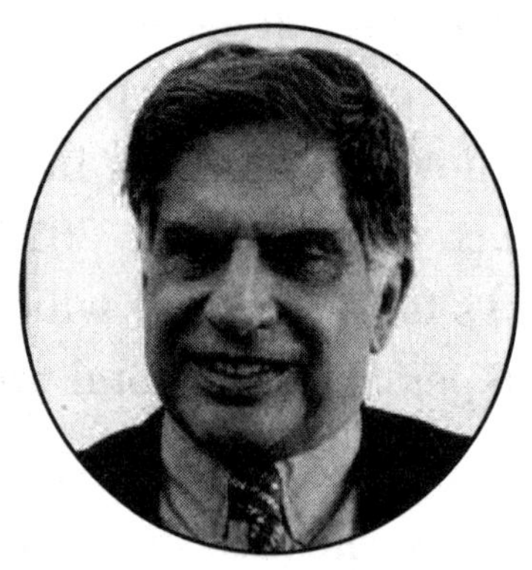

One Century Foils Another Dismissal

Ratan Tata became the chairman of Tata Motors in 1988; absolutely three years before he took the leadership charge of Tata Sons. Since also, the company has been a patromax for Tata to give chances to his bourns. Be it India's first indigenous car (Tata Indica), first SUV (Safari), first micro truck (Ace) or a Rs 1 lakh car for the common public (Nano), Tata Motors has many firsts to its diary.

The accession of Jaguar Land Rover in 2008 catapulted Tata Motors to one of the world's top transport makers. It has also been an unbelievable monetary success. JLR accounts for nearly two-thirds of profit and 90 per cent of consolidated profit. It also helped the company de-risk its finances from the vagrancies of the marketable vehicle business.

The JLR success, in a way, foils Tata Motors' malfunction to coordinate with Indian car buyers, increasingly changing to its rivals. Fixing this will be top priority for Cyrus Mistry, the new chief, given the quantum of fiscal and strategic capital invested by Tata Sons in the company over the times.

According to the Society of Indian Automobile Manufacturers (Siam), Tata Motors' demanding share in the passenger vehicle segment fell to 12.7 per cent during April-November 2012 from 16.4 per cent in 2006-07. It is India's fourth largest passenger car brand, after Maruti Suzuki, Mahindra & Mahindra and Hyundai.

The decelerating in its domestic business is an economic drag. During the 12 months ending September, the domestic business earned just 5.1

per cent operating profit against 12.5 per cent for its consolidated operations. The fiscal rates of the domestic business are indeed worse, with a return on capital employed (RoCE) of just 3.3 per cent in financial year 2012.

Experts are still not losing hope over Tata's apparent failure in the passenger car market. "At best, it accounts for five per cent of the company's consolidated profit and its financial performance is linked to JLR, followed by its commercial vehicle business in India," says the automobile analyst at a leading brokerage company. Further, he adds, success in the home market matters in the long run, as India is set to feature as one of the world's top vehicle markets in the next 10-15 years.

The Cloud-Free Sky

Experts say the company failed to take advantage of preliminary successes. "Tata Motors is an engineering powerhouse and most of its products have been segment builders. Indica was India's diesel hatchback, Sumo started the MPV (multipurpose vehicle) segment, while Safari pioneered SUVs in India but the company failed to carry it forward," says Pradeep Saxena, executive director, TNS India. He finds an incongruity then. "Brand Tata has certain inherent values embodied in it, such as trust, fairness and integrity. The issue is whether these are good enough for the car category or a buyer cares for another set of values such as modernity, innovation and style," he says.

The poor performance in the domestic car market is recognized by the company, particularly by Ratan Tata himself. "Success in the domestic passenger car market is non-negotiable for us. The goal is to become a strong number two in the near term, and eventually target for the market leadership," says the company's spokesperson.

To achieve this, it will first need to restore Tata Motors' brand image and also submerge the market with new products. "A product is a brand in the auto industry and Tata Motors' product line-up is neither exciting enough or known for being sophisticated and stylish. The company's portfolio hasn't changed much in ten years, except routine product refreshments," says a critic. Others blame the Nano failure; the vehicle consumed funds and operation bandwidth for years. However, "If the Nano had clicked and sold as per the company's expectations, Tata Motors would have been the number two car maker by now," says V.G. Ramakrishnan, director of Frost and Sullivan.

The company's invention machine has braked in recent times. In the seven years from 1991 to 1998, Tata Motors launched five different products — Tata Sierra, Estate, Sumo, Safari and Indica. The pace of new launches has slowed significantly and in the last ten years, it launched just four new products — Indica Vista, Indigo Manza, Nano and Aria, besides renovating age-old models.

Action Required

"When the Indica was first launched in 1998, it was competing against the Maruti Zen and Hyundai Santro. The new generation Indica Vista is up against a dozen or more compact cars. The company needs a breakthrough product and not incremental model changes as it has been doing right through," says Pradeep of TNS India.

The company seems to agree. "There has certainly been a quiet period of late (in terms of new product launches). However, there are new products and offerings in the pipeline," it says.

Experts said it might take time but the company had the means, equipment and infrastructure to make a strong revival. "JLR's acquisition distracted the top management for a while but the domestic market will be its top priority now. JLR's success gives Tata Motors the financial muscle and the engineering prowess to adopt an aggressive posture in India," says the auto analyst at a brokerage house here.

If the company makes the comeback, this will be the finest retirement gift from Cyrus Mistry and the company's top operational circuit to Ratan Tata.

❑

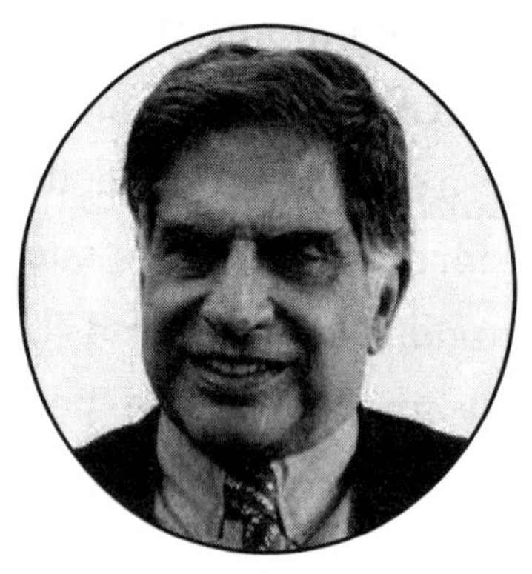

Tata Power: The Global Dimension

Tata Power, the country's largest power mileage in the private sector, would like to forget the year 2012. It had a loss for the first time in over two decades, quite a reversal for a company which not so long ago was a crucial source of growth capital for the entire group. It helped fund the accession of Tata Communications and is a protagonist of the group's telecom adventure, Tata Teleservices. The company remains a heavy megahit in the group, with the third largest balance sheet after Tata Steel and Tata Motors. Ratan Tata became the chairman of Tata Power comparatively late, six years after he became chairman of Tata Sons in 1991.

The company now finds itself during an economic storm, as its biggest investment, on the 4,000 Mw Mundra Ultra Mega Power Design (UMPP) did not go consistent with the intuition. Listed to be completely functional by the middle of the coming year, it will nearly double Tata Power's generating capacity but is rooting a big financial massacre. The total investment in Mundra accounts for nearly a third of the consolidated means.

When the corporate won the shot to develop the Mundra UMPP, to be grounded on imported coal, this was believed to free Tata Power from the constraints of its regulated business that limited returns from its bread-and-butter power distribution and generation business in the Mumbai region. The company hoped to earn better returns from Mundra through husbandry of scale and energy-effective super-critical technology. It had bid assertively, promising to provide power at

₹2.26 a unit. Comparatively, NTPC, the country's largest driver of coal-fired plants, vended power at a normal of ₹2.66 a unit in FY 2012. The government had imaged imported coal-grounded power plants as domestic force was not suitable to embrace the demand.

Tata Power's computations were grounded on plans to import coal from Indonesia when international prices were around $40 a ton at the time of bidding in 2006. It also bought a 30 per cent equity stake in two major Indonesian thermal coal manufacturers, KPC and PTA, in March 2007. But global coal prices surged past $100 a ton in 2011 and the Indonesian government put up an embargo on exports under the labeled price from September 2011. This made import of coal economically unviable for Tata Power and the Mundra planning is now unfit to make indeed functional profit; it cannot service the project debt on its own.

Coastal Gujarat Power Ltd (CGPL), the special purpose vehicle set up to apply the plan, reported operating losses of Rs 2.3 crores on earnings of Rs 363 crores in the quarter ending September. The total loss, including finance and deprecation cost, was Rs 461 crores. In comparison, the Tata Power standalone business reported an operating contour of 27 per cent in the last quarter.

Urging

Cyrus Mistry, the new chairman of the group, now faces the challenge of satisfying Mundra consumers – six devisee state governments – to agree to a price rise so that the project becomes financially feasible.

CGPL is seeking intervention from the Central Electricity Regulatory Commission for an upward modification in rates to over Rs 3 per unit. "We are hopeful of an early resolution of the issue," said Anil Sardana, managing director, Tata Power.

Global rating agency Standard & Poor's has downgraded Tata Power's long-term rating to 'BB -'. This is an academic and non-investment grade rating. "The outlook revision reflects our expectation that Tata Power's cash flow and financial risk profile could deteriorate over the coming six to nine months because the company has breached a debt-to-equity ratio covenant on loans to its Mundra project," S&P

credit analyst Rajiv Vishwanathan observed in a declaration last July.

To alleviate the threat, the company has offered to restructure — it will transfer 75 per cent of its equity interest in Indonesian coal mines to CGPL, so that it uses the dividends from coal to service the debt in the intermediate period.

"To an extent, Tata Power was aware of the risk it was taking on coal prices, so it tried to mitigate it by taking part-ownership of the mines," said Murtuza Arsiwalla, analyst at Kotak Institutional Equities. "But the extreme volatility of coal prices that followed was completely unexpected."

The reversal at Mundra has, still, not dissuaded Tata Power's growth plans or to go laggardly on globalization. It aimed for 26,000 Mw of generation capacity by 2020, by setting up more power plants in India and expanding abroad, to de-risk it from energy dearths and fuel shortage then.

Its non-Mundra business, still, continues to be inflated and is growing at a steady pace. The company enjoys a strong 'AA-' rating standing for its domestic and rupee-denominated borrowing programmes, thanks to its regulated power generation and distribution business. "The rating on Tata Power continues to reflect its strong business position as an integrated power company. Its cash flows from core licensed operations are stable due to the regulated nature of the business," said Amod Khanorkar, analyst with CARE Ratings in a note recently.

❑

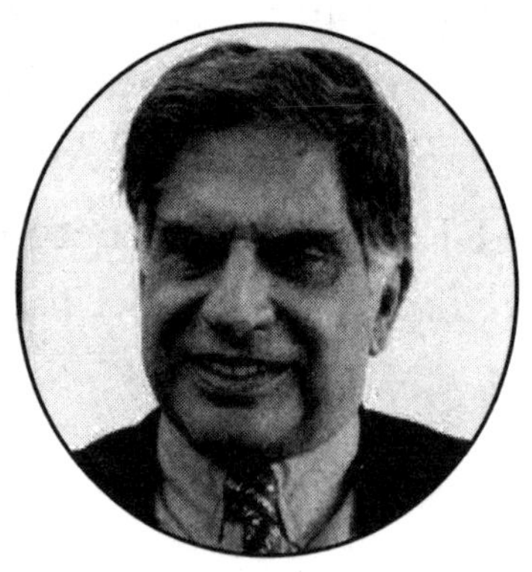

The Defensive Tata

On November 15, 2010, Ratan Tata delivered a lecture on "India in the 21st century: Opportunities and Challenges" in Dehradun, the capital of Uttarakhand. The lecture would have gone overlooked, had Tata not exposed that he thrice tried to get into civil aeronautics but his attempts were unsuccessful because a minister demanded to be paid Rs 15 crores in backhanders and he refused to do so.

"We approached three prime ministers also, but an individual thwarted our efforts to form the airline," he said. "I did not want to go to bed knowing that I set up an airline by paying Rs 15 crores." This demurred up a storm. Some people prompted Tata to name the minister, given the strong anti-corruption statement in the country. Others said there was no point speaking out against the misdemeanour ten years latterly. Yet, it was a rare admission of missed openings in Tata's 20-year-long career as the chairman of Tata Sons.

As he takes stock, Tata will surely feel good about many of his enterprises: the metamorphosis of Tata Steel and Tata Motors, growth of TCS, expansion of Tata Tea, etc. On the other side, his domestic car business has failed to live up to the original pledge of two high-profile launches (the Indica and Nano), he exited FMCG (Tomco and Lakme) and missed the smash, his casing action is still to attain scale, his pharmaceutical incursion (Advinus) is yet to get into the big league, his telecom companies are way behind the leaders, and his aeronautics plans just could not take shape.

J.R.D. Tata had started India's first industrial airline, Tata Airlines, in the 1930s. After Independence, it was nationalized and renamed Air India. Though the Tata group was out of the airline, the business always remained close to its heart. Some days ago, the central government's newer move opened up the opportunity to organize a reunion of J.R.D. Tata's brightest baby, the Air India, to come back home. In the 1990s, when the sector was opened up for classified companies, Tata knew the time had occurred. He snappily put together an alliance with Singapore Airlines to start a domestic carrier. Also the laws changed overnight. Foreign airlines were barred from retaining even a single share in a domestic carrier. Tata's proposed airline with Singapore Airlines could not take off.

Who obstructed the plans?

Maharaj Kishen Kaw, a former mandarin who was the civil aeronautics clerk when Inder Kumar Gujral was the prime minister (April 1997 to March 1998), in his recent book, *An Outsider Everywhere: Revelations by an Insider*, has said that it was the work of Tata's rivals. "The Tatas had mooted a proposal for a private airline with 40 per cent equity contribution from Singapore Airlines. As this would have been a formidable competitor, Jet Airways tried hard to upset rules regarding foreign equity contribution," Kaw wrote. He said that CM Ibrahim, the then civil aviation minister, was not attracted by the Tata offer. "The minister did not clear the file, despite several attempts on my part," Kaw added. The sector, of course, is stuck in fatalities. It is not sure if the stillborn offer was a blessing in disguise.

Telecom is a different story. Tata Teleservices has 76.7 million subscribers (as of October 31, according to the Telecom Regulatory Authority of India), which puts it in the fifth place after Bharti Airtel (186.4 million), Vodafone (153.1 million), Reliance Communications (134 million) and Idea Cellular (115.7 million). Tata Teleservices, earlier had taken the CDMA route, and not GSM, to mobile telephony. Though largely effective for transmitting data, CDMA suffered from some impediments and stumbling blocks. For instance, the handset came whisked with the service. Secondly, a royalty had to be paid to Qualcomm, the service provider, which eroded the gains. The future was with GSM.

The window of occasion to launch GSM service showed up in 2007 when the department of telecommunications, under Andimuthu Raja, decided to arrange GSM spectrum to CDMA players at a consolidated amount for all of India. Effects went crazy for Tata Teleservices right from the launch.

On October 18, Raja, while approving the trade of crossover spectrum noted on the file that "For allocation of spectrum, the date of payment of the required fee should determine the seniority". Three CDMA service operators, Reliance Communications, Shyam Telelink and HFCL Infotel, had applied for the GSM license in 2006. In principles approval was granted to these three on October 18 itself, though the press release to this effect was only issued the following day. On October 19, Reliance Communications deposited the figure of Rs 1,645 crores (for 20 of the 22 telecom circles) and came right on top of the line for spectrum.

It was distributed spectrum on January 10 and 11, 2008. Tata Teleservices applied on October 20. Now, Raja decided to change the policy and conjoined Tata Teleservices with other campaigners of spectrum. In principle he gave approval to Tata Teleservices's offer only on January 10, 2008, when the company was needed to deposit the license amount. Its operations were entered at DoT's reception counter and further delivered to the office of the wireless counsel. Then, the 'ghosts' appeared, and from there the applications went missing!

On December 8, 2010, Tata wrote to Rajeev Chandraskehar, who had alleged of inaptly grabbing spectrum under the crossover window: "The company (Tata Teleservices) has strictly followed the applicable policy and has been severely disadvantaged, as you are well aware, by certain powerful politically connected operators who have willfully subverted policy under various telecom ministers, which has subsequently been regularized to their advantage. The same operators continue to subvert policy, have even paid the fee for spectrum even before the announcement of policy and have 'de facto ownership' in several new telecom enterprises." Tata Teleservices had not got spectrum in Delhi and some other circles even three years after the advertisement of the policy, Tata added.

So, it is hereby clearly understood, that, in telecom, lobbying and political influences are everything.

❑

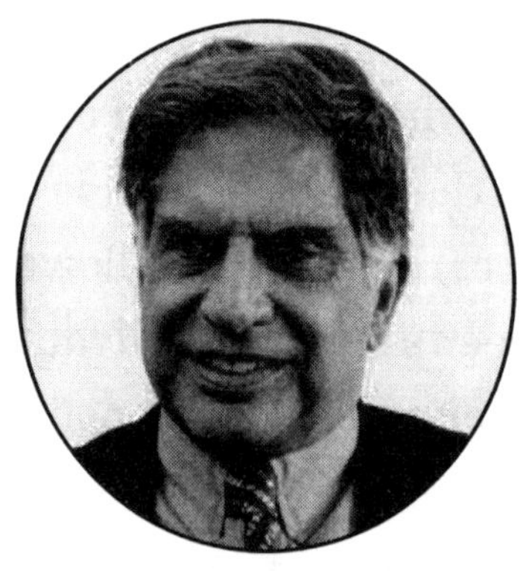

Black Mark in the White Clipboard

Ratan Naval Tata's outstanding career as the master of Tata Sons has seen numerous firsts: high-rattle slugfests were one of them. Right through his two-decade long spell as chairman, Tata has in no way nestled down from any challenger or adversity. Known to speak his mind and that too intimately, he has had several run-sways over the times with peers in commercial India, politicians and, of course, media.

His critics say that Tata was not one to overlook possessions in a rush, and call him bigoted. Rajya Sabha member Rajeev Chandrasekhar says, "The Tata group is caught between trying to maximize return on capital employed like any other business groups in India and remaining rooted to doing business that is immorally comfortable".

Here are the instances of some of his home-ground as well as away-ground hurdles:

1. **Battling the Grey hairs:** Soon after J.R.D. Tata made him the chairman of Tata Industries in 1981, four elderly associates decided that they would make life problematic for Ratan Tata.

   That was perhaps an understatement, as what followed would have put even the worst palace schemes to shame. The battle Tata encountered was from Russi Mody at Tata Steel, Darbari Seth at Tata Chemicals, Ajit Kerkar at Indian Hotels and Nani Palkhivala at ACC – people who ran their companies without any hindrance.

   But Tata delivered a masterstroke — the Tata Sons board gave full support to his offer for administering a rule that set 75 as the retirement age for all Tata directors. While this helped the removal of Seth, ill- health whisked Palkhivala's departure. Ajit Kerkar, who desisted to be the executive chairman of Indian Hotels when he turned 65, was of course banished for different reasons.

It is another matter that Tata himself again changed the retirement rules to continue running the group as the non-executive chairman for another ten springs.

2. **The Telecom Imbroglio:** Telecom has been one of the bitterest hurdles that Tata has overcome. By the time the big bosses – read Tata and Reliance – wanted to get into the business, the nouveau riche were already doing well. From entering the skirmish to selection of technology, Tata fought the GSM atrium tooth and nail. The public slugfest started in 2006, when a commission of the Department of Telecom blazoned its spectrum allocation policy for new technologies like 3G and Wimax. The policy stated that telecom companies would get spectrum depending on the number of consumers they had. With its subscriber base, there was no way that Tata could have aspired

for an advanced share of spectrum compared with the rivals.

So Tata wrote letters to J.S. Sarma, the then secretary, Department of Telecom, and Prime Minister Manmohan Singh, suggesting that the additional spectrum should be auctioned as it was a scarce resource.

Whether it is the matter of out-of-turn spectrum allocation or getting fresh spectrum for free, most of these vexing issues have been raised by Tata at different points. Tata has also admitted that he had a "chemistry problem" with ex-telecom minister Dayandhi Maran.

3. **No Tissue to Confront Issue:** Once the power structure receives its holder, the other equal sectors become inevitable opponents in terms of different means. Like telecom, Tata has fought other business houses even in the power sector. And his anathema in this segment is Anil Ambani's power companies.

   Whether it is the battle for consumers in Mumbai or ultra mega power systems, Tata has used the legal system to fight rivals in this space.

Reliance Infrastructure (erstwhile Reliance Energy) has alleged Tata Power of hooking its guests, while Tata Power sought payment of dues that had collected over a period.

Tata Power has gone to court on the issue of residue coal by Reliance Power from the interned mines that came with the UMPP.

4. **The Singur Turmoil:** This was definitely one of Ratan Tata's biggest despondencies. The Nano project in West Bengal, ended up as a calamity after the Tatas moved out of the state on October 3, 2008, after Mamata Banerjee's Trinamool Congress started the save cropland movement. Tata eventually left Singur, but not before a public disapprobation of the agitation led by Banerjee. Though the court battle over compensation for the Singur land continues, the two protagonists have more recently sought to mend their shattered relationship through pacific tones in their public statements.

5. **The Tape Issue:** What actually put Tata in the eye of the storm were the leaked videotapes that revealed exchanges that his lobbyist and the

proprietor of public relations firm, Vaishnavi Communications, Niira Radia, had with media personnel and government officers. After the videotapes caused a public rampage, Tata said that the leaks were to produce a smokescreen around the 2G contestation. He also moved the Supreme Court, questioning the exposure of private exchanges.

❑

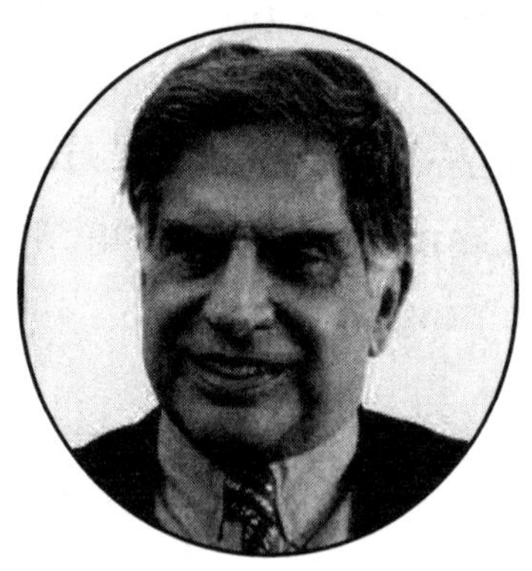

The Global Prospect

It took Ratan Tata a full decade to make the group globalized. But it was the proverbial pause before the storm as what followed was some of the most audacious deals that commercial India had seen till they happened.

The group became bolder as well – Tetley was acquired for $450 million; JLR for $2.3 billion and Corus for $12.1 billion.

"I would put Tata in the larger group of 'globalizing' companies, that is, ones that have an international presence but have still not made their presence felt everywhere in the world. Tata is strong in Britain, the US and South Africa, but less high-profile elsewhere," says Morgen Witzel, author of *Tata: The Evolution of a Corporate Brand*.

In terms of sheer figures, its global operations contributed as much as 58 per cent of the $100 billion (Rs 4.75 lakh crores) group's consolidated earnings in 2011-12. For Tata Steel, the share of global operations is as much as 74 per cent; for Tata Global, it is 70 per cent; for Tata Motors, it is 67 per cent and for Indian Hotels, it is 25.77 per cent.

A snap of the companies, which have gone global, reflect a mixed scenario. The return on net worth (RoNW or return on equity) for Tata Global at 8 per cent is more or less the same at the time of acquiring Tetley and now. In case of JLR, it has leaped from negative to a massive 52 per cent. For Indian Hotels, still, it has declined from 14 per cent to lower than a percentage point. And Tata Steel's RoNW has reduced from 37 per cent to 7 per cent.

In fact, Tata Steel Europe is hurting the group poorly. Indeed Ishat Hussain, non-executive director of Tata Sons, in response to a narrative in the *Economist*, recognized Tata Steel's troubles, "The Return on capital employed (RoCE) since 2010 has been highly distorted by the performance of one business: Tata Steel. The RoCE for Tata companies, excluding Tata Steel Europe and the capital work-in-progress of Tata Steel in India, is 14 per cent."

Evidently, a 4 per cent drag on the overall group's RoCE cannot be taken casually.

Though the fiscal sector extremity since 2008 has led to decelerating down of demand from automobile and construction companies – the key consumers of Corus - many say that the deal was precious. Lakshmi Mittal's $34 billion accession of Arcelor in June 2006 was cheaper at EBITDA (earnings before interest, duty, depreciation and amortization) multiple of 4.3 vis-à-vis 9 for Tata Steel's accession of Corus.

That is reflected in the performance of the share price. When the deal was declared on June 30, 2006, Tata Steel's share price stood at ₹473 and market cap at ₹29,516 crores. In November 2012, the respective figures are ₹377 and ₹37,431 crores. The equity base, still, has increased supremely. To patronize the deal, the group issued 390 million shares, raising the equity base from 580 million to 970 million. During a similar period, the sensex shot up 82 per cent while the company's stock price is down 20 per cent.

The value of the accession has eroded considerably. However, which operates in an analogous terrain, their market cap stands at $26 billion, if one considers peers like Arcelor Mittal. Tata Steel, Europe which has one-fifth of Arcelor Mittal's capacity should be valued at $5 billion. In other words, the market value of Tata Steel is lower than the debt ($6 billion) it raised, and half the overall price paid at $12.1 billion. Indeed capacity utilization has fallen to 14 million tons in FY 2011-12 from 23.1 million tons in FY 07-08.

JLR, on the other hand, is a completely different story; however there were primary interruptions which forced Tata Motors to post a loss of ₹2,465 crores in 2008-09. But now, the marquee automobile company is the crown jewel of the group. In fact, if

JLR had not paid a dividend of ₹1,312 crores to Tata Motors in the second alternate quarter of the current fiscal time, the parent company would have declared a loss.

Within these two giant deals, there is Tetley which has done relatively well. Witzel says, "The Tetley acquisition seems to have gone very well, partly because Tata Beverages has taken a soft approach to managing it. Most people in the UK still don't know that it is possessed by Tata Beverages." And the figures continue to be stable.

Indian Hotels has suffered the mass of a lackluster world economy. "The international acquisitions done by Indian Hotels have not been earning per share accretive due to economic slowdown leading to lower passenger traffic," said Rashes Shah, analyst with ICICI Securities. With the company willing to go aggressive with the Orient Express deal, the results will only show in 10-20 times, say analysts. The figures, as a result, are not too flattering.

While the jury is still out on how Tata has done in his global gambles, the fact is they have been bold, but not inescapably beautiful.

Tata Global Beverages (TGB) may not be big contributors to the Tata kitty, but are still important to its expansion story. Trent, Tata Global Beverages (TGB), Titan Industries and Tata Chemicals have together grown at a compounded annual growth rate of 23 per cent in the past six years. They continue to be the rising stars in the group with each clocking double-number top line growth. Tata Chemicals grew at a CAGR of close to 23 per cent in the last six times. Trent, Titan and TGB grew by 30 per cent, 35 per cent and 13 per cent independently in the same time frame.

While the four companies contributed just about 7 per cent to the total development of the Tata Group in the 2011-12 financial years, critics say this number could go up as these businesses ride the consumption smash.

Group spectators say that the fabulous four have actually helped the over 100-year-old Tata empire mark its presence in daylight sectors similar to fast-moving consumer goods (FMCG), retail, agric, memoir and nano-technology. It is these sectors amongst its other staple sections of information technology, automotive, hospitality, power and steel that the Tatas are highly counting on as they place themselves as an organization of idealism on the global stage.

It is also from among these very sectors that the Tatas' first major international accession happened.

The time was 2000 and the concurrence was Tetley, a company three times the size of TGB also called Tata Tea, with an allocation of 7 per cent of the world tea demand and ranked number two after Unilever's Brooke-Bond-Lipton. TGB was an original player also largely known for tea and coffee products. Its ingrained play was hardly significant beyond Indian props though the company did have a coordinate venture with Tetley for export of its products. But it demanded a strong platform to launch itself on the global stage. That occasion came with the vast amount (Rs. 1,500 crores) of leveraged buyout of Tetley, the largest overseas accession for an Indian company.

While making the advertisement in February 2000, Chairman Ratan Tata had famously said, "It is a bold move and I hope that other Indian corporates will follow."

They did. But more so it gave the Tatas the courage to take on indeed bigger challenges. That is, acquire further businesses across sectors. In Beverages alone in the last decade, TGB has wrapped up a string of deals including Good Earth and Eight O'clock Coffee in the US, Jemca in the Czech Republic and Grand in Russia.

The company retains its appetite for more, but now says that it would like to concentrate on consolidation and organic growth. "We are a natural Beverages company and our focus will be on tea, coffee and water," Harish Bhat, managing director, TGB, had said in a recent interview with *Business Standard.*

The company is open to striking further alliances with like-minded mates, if needed - it has two at the moment, one with PepsiCo, the other with Starbucks - and is keen to increase its earnings from coffee and water.

But TGB is not the only company where Tatas' global intentions have played out ahead of other sectors in the group.

Titan is another case in point. Established as a common venture between the Tatas and the Tamil

Nadu Industrial Development Corporation (TIDCO) in 1984, the company has in the last three decades registered itself not only as a foremost maker of watches in India, but also amongst the pinnacle in the world. It is presently eying the number three position - a jump two places from number five, where it ranks internationally in the watch market.

In India, Titan accounts for about 25 per cent of the volume and 40 per cent of the value of the over 50-million-unit-watch market.

It has also created some adorable brands similar as Fastrack for youth, Raga for women, Nebula, a gold watch targeted at the ultra-expensive customers' end and Sonata at the lower end.

In the last many years, Titan has devoted its attention to other businesses too such as jewellery under Tanishq, which gives it over 70 per cent of its earnings nowadays, and goggles, a new area it ventured into besides leather accessories such as holdalls, belts and bags, as it aims to take advantage of India's consumption and retail smash. Titan's managing director, Bhaskar Bhat, has said that the company will continue looking at all lifestyle accessories barring apparels.

While Titan's growth has been largely driven by organic measures, it has wrapped up many deals like the accession of the Swiss heritage brand Favre-Leuba last time. Enterprise was replete in July this year that it was meaning a $1-billion accession of Canada-grounded luxury watches and jewellery-retailer Harry Winston. But this was negated by the company.

On Trent, the government's move to authorize foreign direct investment in retail has opened up opportunities for a coalition in that part, say analysts. The loss-making company already has a franchise agreement with Tesco under which the Indian firm's Star Bazaar supermarkets use Tesco's supply chains and structure. Both Trent and Tesco are now supposed to be exploring the opportunity of expanding their alliance in the wake of parliament's nod to retail FDI, say sources.

Tata Chemicals, on the other hand, has expanded into three areas: living rudiments, industry rudiments and farm rudiments—from a patron of largely inorganic chemicals such as soda ash, a base component in numerous industries. Under living rudiments come the company's consumer businesses—swab, water, ingrained goods and neutraceuticals. Under industry rudiments, come the core bulk and specialty chemicals and cement, while farm rudiments dwell on crop nutrition and protection and seeds. Company directors say that the metamorphosis from a commodity company to one furnishing complex results in different areas was led by the need to be applicable in changing times. In the last many years, Tata Chemicals has made a series of accessions in inorganic chemicals and has also invested heavily in agribusiness. It is now concentrating its attention on its exploration and development capabilities.

The Nano, master-work of Ratan Tata, has been synonymous with inventions in rising markets. His trouble to fill the white spot between two-wheelers and mini cars for Indian mass family transportation needs has presumably captured the maximum mind space worldwide as an economical engineering success.

The success of Nano was not in just being the cheapest four-wheeler in the world, at Rs 1 lakh at the time of launch. It was the inventions that made the car cheap. The global four-wheeler industry is enthusiastic on modular ways to produce motorcars with different prices and design features. The Nano is erected from modular factors, which can bc made and packed independently for assembly at different locales. In effect, the Nano is designed for distribution in accoutrements assembled and serviced by local entrepreneurs globally.

Germany's Roland Berger Strategy Advisers in its lately-released report on global invention shifting to rising markets, says, "Frugal product inventions must start in the company's mindset", recalling Platonic tune of 'imitation' in other words.

This is what Ratan Tata, outgoing chairman of the $100-billion Tata Group, has been driving in the final half of his captaincy of India's largest business empire for over two decades.

This is also the period when Indian companies saw a rush of global competition in the domestic markets. This made consumers discerning, with better products and enhanced client service.

"With globalization, the need for innovation became more critical for Indian companies' survival," says

Wilfried Aulbur, managing partner, Roland Berger, who co-authored the report with his other associates. "This led many companies to put more focus on innovation to address new market opportunities," he says.

For case, when Korean auto maker Hyundai Motor set up shop in India in 1996, there were five major auto makers in the country: Maruti Udyog (now, Maruti Suzuki India), Hindustan Motors, Premier Automobiles (now, Premier Ltd), TELCO (now, Tata Motors), and Mahindra & Mahindra (M&M).

Now, Hyundai is the second largest auto maker in India after Maruti Suzuki, still leading the pack. Tata Motors and M&M have been in neck-to-neck competition this time for the third and fourth positions.

But the most distinctive part is that Hindustan Motors and Premier Automobiles are nowhere in the race at present, precisely because of their incapability to innovate and upgrade according to the changing market conditions.

Tata Motors had tasted the changing market condition and it brought out the first indigenous four-wheeler, Indica, in 1999; a small truck, the Ace, in 2005 and the innovative Nano in 2008 to capture new market openings. There are more similar exemplifications from the group, similar as setting up Ginger Budget Hotels in 2002 and making a super computer, Eka, in 2005.

In fact, there have been innumerable cases when the over-a-century-old Tata Group has been an avant-garde. In 1907, Tata Steel became the first Indian company to elevate capital in India. J.R.D. Tata founded Tata Airlines in 1932 and TCS in 1968. Tata Motors made India's first indigenous light marketable vehicle, the Tata 407, in 1986.

Though invention, modification and innovation have been in the group's DNA, the urgency for this became more prominent recently. When the economy-marker first opened in the early 1990s, the group realized its business processes were weak. So, in 1995, it introduced the Tata Business Excellence Model. Any company that uses the Tata brand name or totem has to abide by the model. Under this, companies are given scores out of 1000 every time.

But invention within the group was sporadic. "We had to accelerate and create urgency for the democratization of innovation. This had become more important with the Tata Group going global and the Indian economy getting globalized," said Sunil Sinha, CEO of Tata Quality Management Services (a division of Tata Sons) before.

In 2006, an InnoMission (innovation mission) of 10 Tata Group CEOs went to the US and saw invention at work in companies similar as 3M, Microsoft, Intel, Hewlett-Packard and Raytheon. In the coming time, another project was launched, this time in the other direction, to Japanese companies such as Fuji, Olympus, Toshiba, Nissan and Hitachi. A third undertaking went to Cambridge to traverse the eco-system and to find the scope for innovation there.

The first result was the conformation of Tata Group Innovation Forum (TGIF), commanded to act as a catalyst for invention. It meets every two months (in a different area so that native companies can share) to take stock of the situation and omit hindrances.

The coming step was to honour and award invention within the group InnoVista. These awards are locally acclaimed as well as national. Ratan Tata gives the national awards once a time.

There are three categories: Promising Innovations, The Leading Edge and Dare to Try. An independent jury judges the entries. From 101 from 31 companies in 2006, entries rose to 117 from 39 companies in 2007, also to 289 entries from 47 companies in 2008, and from 62 companies in 2009 to entries from 71 Tata companies in 2012.

The sharp leap in entries from 2009 had a lot to do with the triumphant launch of the Nano. "That fired the imagination of the people in the Tata Group," said R. Gopalakrishnan, administrative director at Tata Sons, before.

After much deliberation, TGIF espoused the Innometer developed by Julian Birkinshaw of the London Business School. It measures the invention process and culture on a scale of zero to five, and can be run on the whole company, a unit or even a small platoon.

Another hedge to invention in the group was that the various Tata companies would not communicate with each other. Ratan Tata, when he became chairman in the early 1990s, removed key chieftains like Russi Mody, Ajit Kerkar and Darbari Seth. A group identity was forged, but collaboration still did not take place. So, TGIF decided to set up InnoClusters— groups of companies that could work jointly in diverse areas.

There are four similar clusters: nanotechnology, plastics and mixes, information technology and water. One of the biggest clusters, of 10 companies, is on nanotechnology. "The Swach water purifier is a perfect example where TCS, Tata Chemicals and Titan came together," said Gopalakrishnan.

Further, the TGIF came with a web-grounded open invention action called InnoVerse. Workers can post a problem on the intranet, to which anybody can give an opinion. People can go on ideas with the 1000 karma points they get.

The group spent $2.7 billion on exploration and development in 2010-11, about three per cent of its development in that time. So, has the Tata Group changed? It is still early days, says Gopalakrishnan. "It's not as if there is a storm gathering; it's just some rain here and there."

From a group run by satraps, the outgoing chairman of Tata group, Ratan Tata, will be credited with founding a youthful platoon of CEOs to run their concerned companies, giving them a free hand as long as they followed the introductory principles of ethics, values and commercial governance. Tata hired the best competent talents from across the world as he saw beforehand on that to survive in the wake of profitable liberalization, Indian companies demanded to go global and borrow superlative practices.

Backed by a trusted team A, led by fellow Tata Sons director R.K. Krishna Kumar, Tata led the metamorphosis by handing over unconnected businesses such as cosmetics, detergents and cement — ranking numerous satraps close to precursor J.R.D. Tata. The group rather concentrated on new generation businesses such as telecom, software, retail and cars.

Tata formed a network of youthful CEOs, now in their 40s and running their separate companies efficiently. This includes Karl Slym, hired from General Motors to run Tata Motors after the Nano project was unsuccessful to make a profitable amount of money. There were other youngster fighters as well, such as: Brotin Banerjee, 36, who heads Tata Housing Development Company; N Chandrasekharan, 48,

CEO of TCS; Anil Sardana, 52, of Tata Power; N. Srinath, 49, of Tata Teleservices, and R. Mukundan, 44, CEO of Tata Chemicals.

Although Tata encountered a tough time in his career, thanks to the public fight with Russi Mody and Ajit Kerkar, he managed to ease out the satraps and succeeded in receiving his own people at the rudder of every provision.

According to Tata Group interposers, it was Kumar who was necessary in setting up the race commission for Tata and helped set the retirement age of Tata directors to get around any Russi Mody occasion in future. When Ratan Tata was under siege from Mody, the then chairman of Tata Steel and Kerkar, the then chairman of Indian Hotels, the operators of Taj Hotels, and Darbari Seth of Tata Chemicals, it was Kumar who played an important part in the ouster of the satraps.

Since also, Tata and Kumar have led the transition of the group from a regulatory set up to a nimble-footed group, which is now earning half of its $100-billion earnings from its overseas operations. In a recent interview with *Business Standard*, Kumar said the aggressive combinations and accessions policy of the group is now eventually giving dividends. "Just look at the JLR; we are now earning every quarter what we spent on buying the company," he said. In 2012, JLR made an over-profit on a profit of about Rs 1.16 lakh crores.

In Tata Chemicals, R. Mukundan is navigating the company towards specialty chemicals and consumer products, as customers insist on change along with increasing expenditure. "As India becomes more urbanized and as income situations and habits change, the country's GDP will rise and supply chains will shift; there will be demand for new types of chemicals and products," says Mukundan. As Tata Steel Managing Director H.M. Nerurkar is due to retire beforehand coming time, interposers say a hunt is already on for the coming MD. Among the frontal runners is 44-year-old Kaushik Chatterjee, the CFO of Tata Steel, who helped the company restructure its debt taken to fund its accession abroad of Corus.

As Kumar is also retiring from Tata Sons and group companies by July coming time, Tata's new chairman Cyrus Mistry will be starting his innings with a fresh line up. This will help the new chairman to make his own platoon. With Tata promising every help to his successor, it will be now over to Mistry to take the Tata Group to a better and more profitable extent.

❑

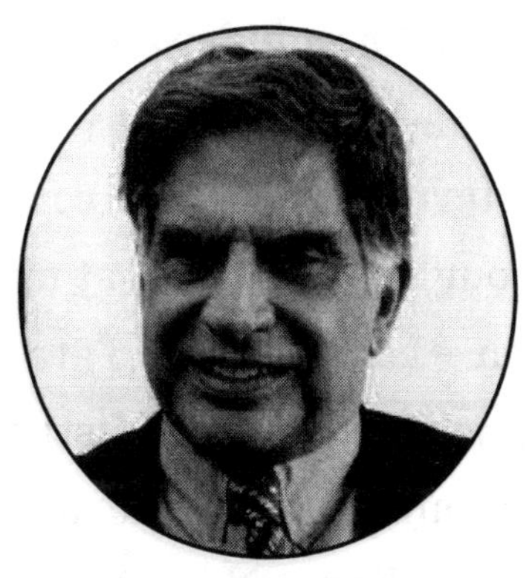

The Relay Race Continues

In August 2010, Ratan Tata announced that he would be retiring as the group chairman in December 2012. He earlier already took retirement in 2012 from all the executive positions he had been into abide by the group's retirement policy of announcing it at the age of 65. He was at the age of his official retirement in 2007 (when he turned 70 years), but the board of Tata Sons modified the policy and extended the retirement age of non-executive directors to 75 years that permitted him to continue as the head of the Tata group.

Over the years, when talking about his retirement, Ratan Tata had said he would prefer a person in his 40s or early 50s to replace him as that would give the new chairman a long term. To avoid the contradictions that he had to go through in 1991, he set up a five-member hunt commission – consisting of Tata Sons directors, R.K. Krishna Kumar and Cyrus Mistry, who is the son of Shapoorji Pallonji Mistry, the largest individual shareholder in Tata Sons; Noshir Soonawala, former vice chairman of Tata Sons; Shirin Bharucha, group legal counsel and Warwick University Professor, Lord Kumar Bhattacharyya – to find the group's coming chairman. The commission was given an open accreditation to find the right seeker, who could be within or outside the Tata group, an Indian public or a non-Indian. Several known names were considered, with Noel Tata, being acceptable by many as the likely victor. Noel Tata was not only Ratan Tata's half-brother, but also Shapoorji Pallonji Mistry's son-in-law. He was the Vice Chairman of Trent Ltd. and the Managing Director of Tata International.

Anyway, the commission which had primarily set itself a deadline of March 2011 to find a successor attempted to find a suitable and competent seeker. R.K. Krishna Kumar said, “Our committee has come to the conclusion that we cannot find a replacement for Mr. Tata! We may have to change and rearrange the model in terms of what we are looking for. It is not an easy task, but we will identify the next chairman of Tata Sons within a few weeks by the end of May or early June.”

Eventually, on November 23, 2011, the hunt commission recommended Cyrus Mistry, its former member who had recued himself from the commission in early 2011, as the coming Tata group chairman. Mistry, an alumnus of Imperial College, London (Engineering), and London Business School (Management), had been a member of the board of Tata Sons since 2006.

Describing the choice as a “good and far-sighted one”, Ratan Tata said, “I have been impressed with the quality and calibre of his participation, his astute observations and his humility. Don’t be fooled by his quiet demeanour. He is his own person, knows where he wants to be. I feel confident that he will lead the group in a manner that is of the highest quality. Cyrus is the right person for the job, I welcome him."

Though this selection could not avoid the difficulties in acceptance as the social media and virtual world had a significant impact not only on professional agenda but on personal aspects too. Dismissing sundries that his larger-than-life persona would prevaricate or temporize after he retired, Ratan Tata said, "I don't think it is right to have a ghost to shadow over somebody" and his advice to Mistry was, "you should be your own person, you should take your own call and you should decide what you want to".

Accepting the responsibility, Cyrus Mistry said, "...the responsibility of Chairmanship brings with it the winds of change, but the core of the Tata Group must and will remain unchanged. Our commitment to maintaining the highest ethical standard in the conduct of our enterprises; our continuous emphasis on business excellence and managerial competence; our belief in our employees and their well-being; our sense of obligation to the customers we serve; our responsibilities towards the environment and the communities that we touch and the greater good of the countries we operate in – without this core DNA that is uniquely Tata, there is nothing to differentiate us from our peers.

The Tata Group's revenue today stands at over $100 billion. That seems an incredible figure when you consider where we were a decade ago. With our collaborative zeal and effort, I am convinced that we can together write a future that continues to build on the past and takes the Tata name to newer frontiers of growth. "

❑

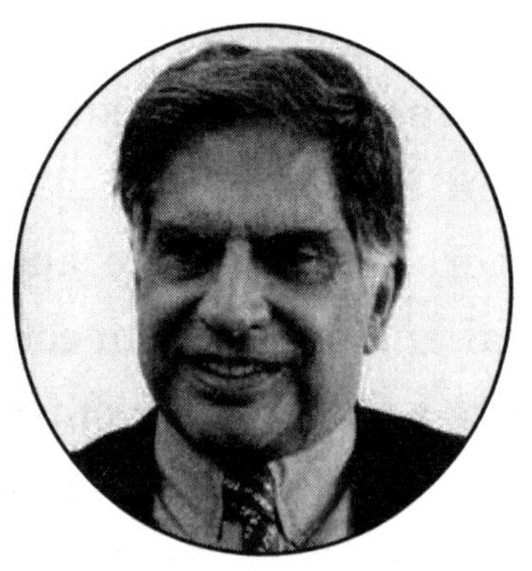

The Policy Differs, Not the Kingdom, Nor The King

Unlike his precursor, J.R.D. Tata, who in 1991 handed over to him the chairmanship of Tata Sons as well as control of the trusts, Ratan Tata will continue to retain control of the second. It is noteworthy, that, there is no retirement age at the trusts, which together control around 66 per cent of the shares of Tata Sons.

But what will keep Tata really busy in his new office at Elphinstone Building are his mega plans for the trusts, which so far attracted only half his attention. The first suggestion of that came in his acceptance speech for a Lifetime Achievement Award introduced by the Rockefeller Foundation when he said his "life's work isn't done yet" as he has not been able to touch multitudes at the bottom of the class structure in society.

Tata easily believes "patchwork philanthropy" — giving a bit of cloth here and food there — would not go far. So he had moved down relatively beforehand from a donator-dependent model from a cooperation model. The alternate part of that drive would come now as Tata does not follow the common belief that charitable institutions have to operate on a hay budget and does not need to produce a professionally-run commercial body.

In a recent interview to American TV intelligencer Charlie Rose, Tata laid out at least a part of his blue-print. He said that he would concentrate on pastoral development, conservation of water and his most important aim is to do better in nutrition for children and pregnant women.

That is a long enough list. But does it mean he would cut himself off absolutely from all that is ever considered marketable in nature? The answer is a big No. Just like JRD, he would remain Chairman Emeritus of Tata Sons and a number of other associate group companies – an ornamental designation — but one which provides him the moral authority to offer advice if asked for by the new Chairman. Tata himself has made it clear that he would be available to anyone seeking his advice but would refrain from taking any active part in the handling of the group's businesses.

Going by the extraordinary closeness he shares with Cyrus Mistry, the latter would not be abashed or hesitate in seeking his counsel. The advice would clearly be much more frequent in matters relating to Tata Motors. The company, which is absolutely closest to Tata's heart, is suddenly feeling the pressure from newer challengers like Mahindra & Mahindra because of an indifferent performance in domestic markets. Tata has also made no secret desire to remain engaged with the Nano. Going by his public statements, Tata would obviously attempt to reverse that indeed after he retires as he has himself said he would like to be "involved" instead of plan-chalking this is often the position that Nano deals can be. And also there is the buzz about Tata planning to set up a transnational centre with state-of-the-art installations to design a wide range of products. The project centre would be relatively close to his heart as Tata has often said that the one benefit of studying in the School of Architecture was that it tutored him to fiddle when exhausted. He said board meetings were one place he would get tired – that coercion, thankfully, has just got over.

All this is quite a sprinkle for people too junior in age and in the florescence of their working life. But Tata would do some extra. For instance, he has formerly said he would like to attend the annual general meetings of Tata group companies as a shareholder and ask questions. Further, Tata will continue to be on the board of directors of Alcoa, apart from being on the international advisory boards of Mitsubishi, the American International Group, JP Morgan Chase, Rolls Royce, Temasek Holdings and the Monetary Authority of Singapore. He is also on the board of trustees of Cornell University and the University of Southern California.

❑

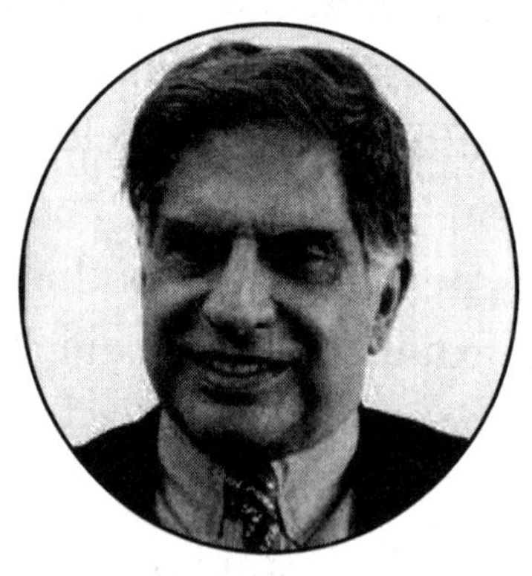

The Fantasy Breakdown

In one of the most dramatic incidents in recent history, the board of directors of Tata Group on October 24, 2016 suggested for the retrenchment of its chairman Cyrus Mistry with immediate effect and made Ratan Tata the interim chairman, and in February 2017, Mistry was removed as a chairman for Tata Sons. The National Company Law Appellate Tribunal (NCLAT) had decided in December 2019 that the removal of Cyrus Mistry as the Chairman of Tata

Sons was illegal and that he should be restored. India's Supreme Court heard an appeal by the $111-billion Empire to quash the NCLAT order that directed the Tata group to rehire the man it fired as chairman. Ratan Tata is tête-à-tête leading the charge in the case, and filed a separate solicitation challenging the ruling in the Supreme Court. The Supreme Court has stayed the NCLAT order that permitted Cyrus Mistry to be restored as Tata Sons' chairman in January 2020. Still the Supreme Court upheld the redundancy of Cyrus Mistry. Ratan Tata made a comeback, taking over the company's interim master for four months. On January 12, 2017, Natarajan Chandrasekharan was suggested as the chairman of Tata Sons, a step he assumed in February 2017.

❑

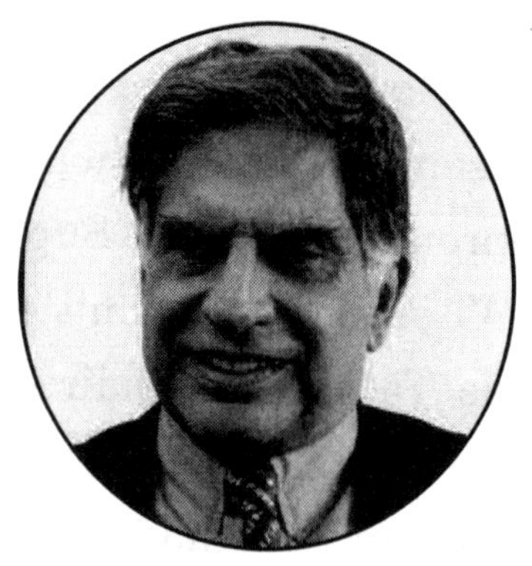

The Marks Unmarked

Ratan Tata had to face public embarrassment in 2010 when his private exchanges with Niira Radia got publicized on the electronic media. Next time he had to lose face was when the Tata Group forced Cyrus Mistry to abdicate as Chairman, presumably at the asseveration of Ratan Tata. Critics said, ironically, Ratan Tata had brought Cyrus Mistry as his successor with considerable fanfare. Apart from these two difficulties, professional life of Ratan

Tata has been without any mark. He has in no way been plant deficient in his conduct as Chairman of the Tata Group or earlier as hand of the Tata Group companies.

❑

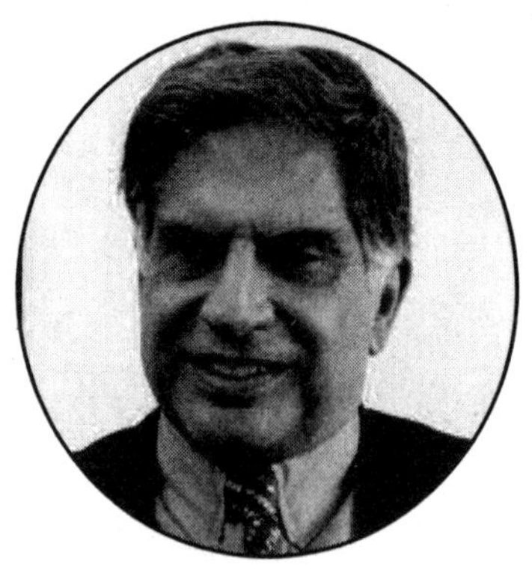

The Current Perusal

Tata invested personal savings in Snapdeal – one among India's leading e-commerce websites – and, in January 2016, Teabox, a web premium Indian tea seller, and CashKaro.com, a reduction coupons saver and cash-back website. He has made small investments in both early and late stage companies in India, like Rs 0.95 crores in Ola Cabs. In April 2015, it was reported that Tata had acquired a stake in Chinese smartphone company Xiaomi. In 2016, he invested in Nestaway, a web portal to seek out fully furnished flats for bachelors who later acquired Zenify to start out family rental segment and online pet care portal, Dogspot. Tata Motors unraveled the primary batch of Tigor Electric Vehicles from its Sanand Plant in Gujarat, regarding which Ratan Tata said, "Tigor indicates a willingness to fast-forward India's electric dream. The government has set an ambitious target to possess only electric cars by 2030."

❑

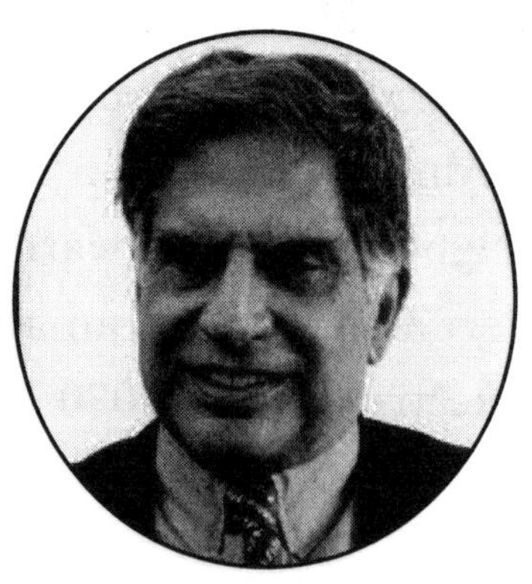

Philanthropist Tata

Tata is a strong devotee of education, pharmaceuticals and rural development, and considered as one of the leading philanthropists in India. Tata backed-up the University of New South Wales Faculty of Engineering to develop capacitive deionization to supply better water to marginal areas.

Tata Hall at the University of California, San Diego (UC San Diego), opened in November 2018, offers facilities for the biological and physical sciences and is the home of the Tata Institute for Genetics and Society. The Tata Institute for Genetics and Society, although a bi-national institution, coordinates the research-programme between UC San Diego and research operations in India to help in societal and infrastructure development within the area of battling vector-borne diseases. Tata Hall is known as in recognition of a generous $70 million from Tata Trusts.

Tata Education and Development Trust, a humanitarian undertaking of Tata Group, endowed a $28 million Tata Scholarship Fund which will allow Cornell University to supply aid to undergraduate students from India. The scholarship fund will support approximately 20 scholars at any given time and can ensure that the absolute best Indian students to get access to Cornell, irrespective of their financial conditions. The scholarships are going to be awarded annually; recipients will have the opportunity of the scholarship for the duration of their undergraduate study at Cornell.

In 2010, Tata Group companies and Tata charities donated $50 million for the development of an executive centre at Harvard Business School

(HBS). The head quarter has been named Tata Hall, after Ratan Tata (AMP '75), chairman emeritus of Tata Sons. The entire construction costs are estimated at $100 million. Tata Hall is founded within the northeast corner of the HBS campus, and is dedicated to the Harvard Business School's mid-career Executive Education programme. It is seven storeys tall, and about 155,000 gross square feet. It houses approximately 180 bedrooms, additionally to academic and multi-purpose spaces.

Tata Consultancy Services (TCS) has given the loftiest ever donation by a corporation to Carnegie Mellon University (CMU) for a facility to research in cognitive systems and autonomous vehicles. TCS donated $35 million for this grand 48,000 square-foot building that is called TCS Hall.

In 2014, Tata Group endowed the Indian Institute of Technology, Bombay and formed the Tata Centre for Technology and Design (TCTD) to develop design and engineering principles and equipment suited to the requirements of individuals and communities with limited resources. They gave ₹950 million to the institute which was the highest ever donation received in its history.

Tata Trusts, under the Chairmanship of Ratan Tata, provided a grant of ₹750 million to the Centre for Neuroscience, Indian Institute of Science to review mechanisms determining the causes, symptoms for Alzheimer's disease and to evolve methods for its early diagnosis and treatment. This grant was to be propagated 5 years starting in 2014.

Tata Group, under the leadership of Ratan Tata, formed the MIT Tata Centre of Technology and Design at Massachusetts Institute of Technology (MIT) with a mission to deal with the challenges of resource-constrained communities, with a primary specialization in India.

❑

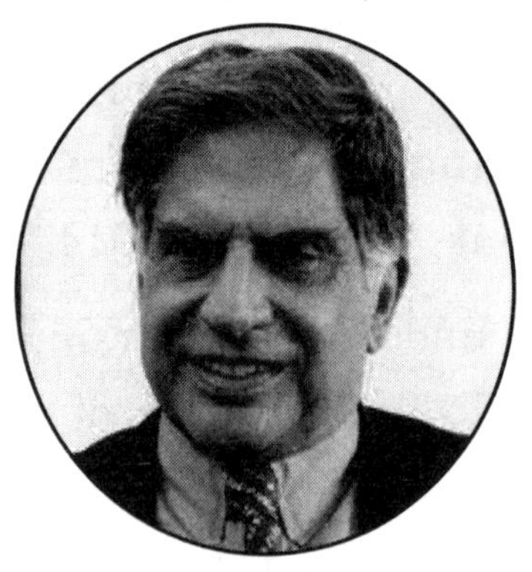

A Successful Leader

The leadership style of Ratan Tata is deeply embedded in Indian morality. Ratan Tata served the Tata Group for nearly 50 years. He has been relatively active indeed after relinquishing his position as Chairman of the Tata Group in 2012. He is now focusing on the charitable arms of the Tata Group. Infact, he has also turned an angel investor and adroit capital financier. He has supported a number of launch-ups in recent history. Ratan Tata has also been awarded the Padma Vibhushan (2008) and Padma Bhushan (2020)—the Government of India's third and alternate loftiest civilian awards.

Several factors have made Mr. Tata what he is now; some of his Success Mantras are:

1. **Conforming to Life:** Mr. Tata though born and raised in an illustrious family, saw what no child should see, i.e. separation of his parents. Yet he acclimatized well growing up with his grandparents. While he was in the US, he did not live a lavish life. On his return to India, he understood the value of the occasion to take part in the family business, when J.R.D. Tata insisted that he should not return abroad, giving up his intentions in a way to continue his dream job at IBM. Latterly, after having made NELCO a profit-making unit, all the loss-making units were transferred to him. The world saw the mastery of Mr. Tata when all the loss-making companies handed over to him started performing well. He has proved that in the course of life, there are numerous ups and downs. The need, still, is to snappily acclimatize to those changes and make

the best out of oneself and the situation, to bring success and passion in the pursuit of life.

2. **Morality:** Mr. Tata was raised by his grandmother, and she indoctrinated a sense of discipline in him. J.R.D. Tata saw this efficiency in practice yielding good consequences. Therefore, he was made the chairman in 1991. Still, also Tata Group would have been in decline, if he were a man of casual attitude and flexible principles. For instance, when Bill Ford tried to affront Mr. Tata, he was determined to take sweet vengeance by proving to the world that Tata Motors demanded no mercy. This negative occasion of his life further strengthened him in no way to vend out any Tata unit; for this, he ensured that the best practices were followed among the workers and employers.

3. **Good Will and Determination:** Mr. Tata always took pride in the heritage of his group. He never displayed any pride or showed off what he has got. He is a lone man with no family and lives with two dogs, offers sanctum to slapdash dogs in bad rainfall. This is the good will that he

carries with himself. In every testing or grueling time in his life, he has never given up, and the result is, under his term of chairmanship earnings grew 40 pack and profit by 50 times. If one can learn from him not to give up and keep following the integral path of good will in particular and professional life, finally its results can be phenomenal.

4. **Thinking for Workers:** The Tata Group and Mr. Tata especially, always understood that workers could make or break the company. They offer their diligence, time, energy, and enthusiasm because of which the group functions. Therefore, one reason for his success is the fact that when it comes to offering gratuities and weal to workers, they follow the most excellent practices. It is to the extent to maintain satisfaction and happiness situations in them to ensure the best productivity rates. It fulfills the integral aspect of running the Tata Group, i.e. broader philanthropic weal through a qualitative change in people's lives.

5. **Learning from the West:** Mr. Tata followed the principle that worked the best for Tata Group, i.e. learning from the West. Mr. Tata was

apprehensive in the post-liberalization period and rising privatization, the competition would come through the channels of globalization. He ensured that the best wisdom and technology was used to intensify camaraderie and produce quality products. He invested heavily on the subject of invention and it is this subject that has driven the change under the period of Mr. Tata making him all the way more successful, so much that today every Indian takes pride to enjoy the luxury and comfort of a five star rated Global NCAP buses, which is over and further all the safety parameters of security quested by the Government of India.

❑

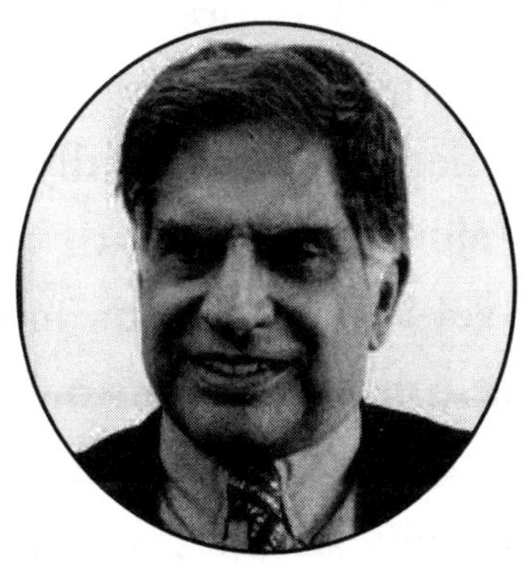

Final Words

The mission and aim of the Tata group has always been to advance India's progress by new and modernized means and introduction of technological support through industrialization. Whenever the dictator changes, people were sure that the reign would not change, as every chairperson will continue the former's legacy through efficiency and competence. Ratan Tata, the iconic maestro, was no exception. Right from facing challenges at initial stages to handle the hurdles aroused from home-grounds, making the in-house persons convinced to expand the business worldwide, following the glorious paths of his superlative precursors like Jamsetji Tata, R.D. Tata and obviously his favourite Jeh (J.R.D. Tata). He not only successfully carried forward the baton; he rejuvenated it with new ornaments and set up a velvet-turf for his upcoming successors, creating a pinnacle of glory in his own hand. Even if he does not actively play a role, abiding by the strict rules and regulations of Tata group, his umbrella will always be there to encourage and take India industrially to the golden gate of paradise.

❑

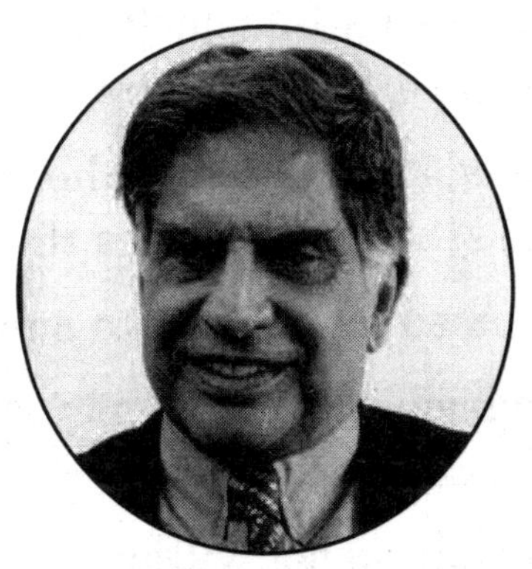

Top Motivational Quotes By Ratan Tata

1. Always deliver more than expected.
2. Apart from values and ethics which I have tried to live by, the legacy I would like to leave behind is a very simple one - that I have always stood for what I consider to be the right thing, and I have tried to be as fair and equitable as I could be.
3. At Tatas, we believe that if we are not among the top three in an industry, we should look seriously

at what it would take to become one of the top three players or think about exiting the industry.

4. Banana republics are run on cronyism.
5. Britain needs a real push. It needs nationalism. The sort of spirit that appears during a war.
6. Business needs to go beyond the interest of their companies to the communities they serve.
7. Challenges need to be given to an organization.
8. Chase the vision, not the money, the money will end up following you.
9. Companies that do not will undoubtedly die.
10. Don't play games that you don't understand, even if you see lots of other people making money from them.
11. Don't take too much advice. Most people who have a lot of advice to give — with a few exceptions — generalize whatever they did. Don't over-analyse everything.
12. Every time we launch a feature, people shout at us.
13. Everyone thinks only about his profit.
14. Get big quietly, so you don't tip off potential competitors.
15. Governance is an important thing, not an application where it suits one so, to micro-control where it suits them on the other hand.

16. Having said that, I hope that a hundred years from now we will spread our wings far beyond India.
17. I admire very successful people. But if that success has been achieved through too much ruthlessness, then I may admire that person, but I can't respect him.
18. I am proud of my country. But we need to unite to make a unified India, free of communalism and casteism.
19. I came seriously close to getting married four times, and each time I backed off in fear or for one reason or another. Each occasion was different, but in hindsight when I look at the people involved, it wasn't a bad thing what I did. I think it may have been more complex had the marriage taken place.
20. I do not know how history will judge me, but let me say that I've spent a lot of time and energy trying to transform the Tatas from a patriarchal concern to an institutional enterprise.
21. I don't believe in taking right decisions.
22. I followed someone who had very large shoes. He had very large shoes. Mr. J.R.D. Tata. He was a legend in the Indian business community. He had been at the helm of the Tata organization for 50 years. You were almost starting to think he was going to be there forever.

23. I have always been very confident and very upbeat about the future potential of India. I think it is a great country with great potential.

24. I have been constantly telling people to encourage people, to question the unquestioned and not to be ashamed to bring up new ideas, new processes to get things done.

25. I have two or three cars that I like, but today, Ferrari would be the best car I have driven in terms of being an impressive car.

26. I may have hurt some people along the way, but I would like to be seen as somebody who has done his best to do the right thing for any situation and not compromised.

27. I take decisions and then make them right.

28. I think the environment has become more competitive. That has made the Indian industry more concerned with a) its customers, b) the quality of its products, and c) its brand image in the marketplace.

29. I think the Tata Group's greatest contribution to the growth of the Indian economy and Indian industry probably happened in the pre-independence era.

30. I think there are many honest businessmen.

31. I think you can have certain specific rules for engaging with India... for example, not allowing mineral resources to be taken out of the country... but there is not a shred of doubt in my mind that

when you open an economy you should do it in totality.

32. I will certainly not join politics.
33. I would like to be remembered as a clean businessman who has not partaken in any twists and turns beneath the surface, and one who has been reasonably successful.
34. I would say that one of the things I wish I could do differently would be to be more outgoing.
35. I, for one, am not the kind who loves dwelling on the 'I'.
36. Ideas are easy. Implementation is hard.
37. If history remembers me at all, I hope it will be for this transformation.
38. If it stands the test of public scrutiny, do it... if it doesn't stand the test of public scrutiny then don't do it.
39. If people like you, they'll listen to you, but if they trust you, they'll do business with you.
40. If there are challenges thrown across, then some interesting, innovative solutions are found. Without challenges, the tendency is to go on the same way.
41. If you are not embarrassed by the first version of your product, you've launched too late.

42. If you want to walk fast, walk alone. But if you want to walk far, walk together.
43. If you're interested in the living heart of what you do, focus on building things rather than talking about them.
44. If your actions inspire others to dream more, learn more, do more and become more, you are a leader.
45. India has probably lost its position to China as the world's workshop. At the same time, it has the power to be ahead of China when it comes to knowledge. Not that the Chinese are far behind. They will get there.
46. Indian car buyers have not been exposed to customer care in a competitive environment.
47. IT and the entire communications business have the greatest growth potential. But if you're talking about sheer size, the steel and auto industries will remain at the top.
48. It needs people really to want to see the UK sitting again, maybe not as a colonial power, but as an economic power.
49. It would, therefore, be a mark of failure on my part if it were perceived that Ratan Tata epitomizes the Group's success.
50. It's not about ideas. It's about making ideas happen.

51. I've never believed protectionism of that kind will lead us anywhere.

52. Jardine is the largest dealer of Mercedes in the world. They also sell cars for two or three Japanese makers.

53. Make every detail perfect and limit the number of details to perfect.

54. Modesty is necessary, even if there is also a need for a certain amount of national pride. When it comes down to it, we have managed our country's economy poorly for long enough.

55. My concern is that the government doesn't appear to care about manufacturing.

56. No one can destroy iron, but its rust can! Likewise, no one can destroy a person, but its mindset can!

57. Nothing works better than just improving your product.

58. One hundred years from now, I expect the Tatas to be much bigger than it is now. More importantly, I hope the Group comes to be regarded as being the best in India... best in the manner in which we operate, best in the products we deliver and best in our value systems and ethics.

59. One of the weaknesses of the Indian industry is that in many areas... like consumer goods... it is

very fragmented. Individually, companies might not be able to survive.

60. Our challenge is to invest sufficiently in education.
61. People of great power wield great power, but people of lesser power or people who have fallen out of power go to jail without adequate evidence, or their bodies are found in the trunks of cars.
62. People still believe what they read is necessarily the truth.
63. Power and wealth are not two of my main stakes.
64. Some foreign investors accuse us of being unfair to shareholders by using our resources for community development. Yes, this is money that could have made for dividend payouts, but it also is money that's uplifting and improving the quality of life of people in the rural areas where we operate and work. We owe them that.
65. Some people dream of success, while other people wake up every morning and make it happen.
66. Take the stones people throw at you, and use them to build a monument.
67. The country is now universally recognized as a nation on the move and takes its place amongst the successful economies in the region.
68. The day I am not able to fly will be a sad day for me.
69. The early Rockefellers made their wealth from being in certain businesses and remained personally very wealthy. Tata's were different

in the sense the future generations were not so wealthy. They were involved in the business but most of the family wealth was put into the trust and most of the family did not enjoy enormous wealth.

70. The fastest way to change yourself is to associate with people who are already the way you want to be.

71. The foreign investment adds a sense of competition; we should see this as a wake-up call to modernize and upgrade.

72. The future potential is enormous but the country's destiny is in our hands.

73. The government should do its job. The government's job is to run the country, to manage the country, to govern the country.

74. The Group's investments in industries such as steel, textiles, power and hotels were certainly driven by an entrepreneurial spirit, but they were driven, even more, I think, by a desire to make India self-sufficient and independent of its colonial masters then.

75. The political system of the People's Republic of China can make things easy. Decisions are made quickly and results come quickly, too. In our democracy (in India), on the other hand, such things are extremely difficult.

76. The strong live and the weak die. There is some bloodshed, and out of it emerges a much leaner industry, which tends to survive.

77. The Telco is committed to commercial vehicles, where it is bound to remain a major player. What may well happen in the future is we may split the company into two business units.

78. The time has come for performance to be measured and for allocated funds of the government to reach the people for whom they were intended.

79. The time has come to move from small increments to bold, large initiatives.

80. The time has come to stretch the envelope and set goals which were earlier not seen to be possible.

81. The value of an idea lies in using it.

82. There are many things that, if I have to relive, maybe I will do it another way. But I would not like to look back and think about what I have not been able to.

83. There is no reason to now think that we can conquer the world.

84. Ups and downs in life are very important to keep us going because a straight line even in an ECG means we are not alive.

85. We can be a truly great nation if we set our sights high and deliver to the people the fruits of continued growth, prosperity and equal opportunity.

86. We have provinces, we have the rule of law, and we have a system of justice. But those are also weaknesses when compared with China. On the other hand, one of our strengths is that we are very individualistic, and as individuals, we are very creative. But that, too, is a weakness, because it keeps us from working well together.

87. We like to say that India has the advantage of being a large market.

88. We live in a highly competitive world and we Indians have to struggle to catch up.

89. We need to build India into a land of equal opportunities for all.

90. We need to stop taking baby steps and start thinking globally. It seems to be helping.

91. We're responsible for the fortunes of the company but this is a bone-dry situation in terms of access to credit. Nobody can operate on that basis unless you have large cash balances, which we don't.

92. What are the crumple zones on scooters? The helmet is the only crumple zone I can think of.

93. What do you need to start a business? Three simple things: know your product better than anyone, know your customer, and have a burning desire to succeed.

94. What I have done is to establish growth mechanisms, play down individuals and play up the team that has made the companies what they are.

95. What I would like to do is to leave behind a sustainable entity of a set of companies that operate in an exemplary manner in terms of ethics, values and continue what our ancestors left behind.

96. What is needed is a consortium of companies in one industry, presenting a strong front to the multinationals. The Swiss watch industry did this.

97. When you find an idea that you just can't stop thinking about, that's probably a good one to pursue.

98. When you see in places like Africa and parts of Asia abject poverty, hungry children and malnutrition around you, and you look at yourself as being people who have well-being and comforts, I think it takes a very insensitive, tough person not to feel they need to do something.

99. Wonder what your customer wants? Ask. Don't tell.

100. Young entrepreneurs will make a difference in the Indian ecosystem.

❑

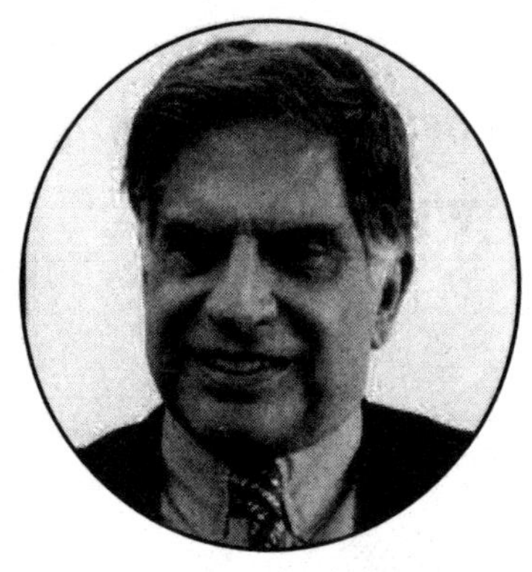

Bibliography

1. Ratan Tata Legacy—An eBook Compilation of reports published in *Business Standard* (dated: December 8, 2012, December 24, 2012, December 25, 2012, December 26, 2012, December 27, 2012, December 28, 2012).
2. *Leading the Tata Group* (A): *The Ratan Tata Years*, by K.S. Manikandan, K. Rajyalakshmi and J. Ramachandran.

3. *Infallibility of Ratan Tata: A Case Study* by Shweta Jha.

4. *Success Principles of Ratan Tata* by Abhishek Kumar.

5. *Beyond the Last Blue Mountains* by R.M. Lala.

6. *Ratan Tata*_Wikipedia.

❑